Medical Illness
and Schizo

Medical Illness and Schizophrenia

Edited by

Jonathan M. Meyer, M.D.

Henry A. Nasrallah, M.D.

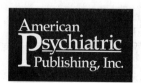

American Psychiatric Publishing, Inc.

Washington, DC
London, England

Note: The authors have worked to ensure that all information in this book is accurate at the time of publication and consistent with general psychiatric and medical standards, and that information concerning drug dosages, schedules, and routes of administration is accurate at the time of publication and consistent with standards set by the U. S. Food and Drug Administration and the general medical community. As medical research and practice continue to advance, however, therapeutic standards may change. Moreover, specific situations may require a specific therapeutic response not included in this book. For these reasons and because human and mechanical errors sometimes occur, we recommend that readers follow the advice of physicians directly involved in their care or the care of a member of their family.

Books published by American Psychiatric Publishing, Inc., represent the views and opinions of the individual authors and do not necessarily represent the policies and opinions of APPI or the American Psychiatric Association.

Copyright © 2003 American Psychiatric Publishing, Inc.
ALL RIGHTS RESERVED

Manufactured in the United States of America on acid-free paper
07 06 05 04 03   5 4 3 2 1
First Edition

Typeset in Baskerville.

American Psychiatric Publishing, Inc.
1000 Wilson Boulevard
Arlington, VA 22209-3901
www.appi.org

Library of Congress Cataloging-in-Publication Data
Medical illness and schizophrenia / edited by Jonathan M. Meyer, Henry A. Nasrallah.—1st ed.
    p. ; cm.
    Includes bibliographical references and index.
    ISBN 1-58562-106-4 (alk. paper)
    1. Schizophrenics—Diseases. 2. Schizophrenics—Medical care. 3. Mentally ill—Diseases 4. Mentally ill—Medical care. I. Meyer, Jonathan M., 1962– II. Nasrallah, Henry A.
    [DNLM: 1. Schizophrenia—complications. 2. Schizophrenia—epidemiology. 3. Comorbidity. 4. Patient Care. WM 203 M489 2003]
    RC514.M425 2003
    616'.0087'4—dc21

                                                        2003044381

British Library Cataloguing in Publication Data
A CIP record is available from the British Library.

Contents

Contributors

Alan Berkman, M.D.

Assistant Professor of Epidemiology, Mailman School of Public Health, Columbia University, New York, New York

Daniel E. Casey, M.D.

Associate Director of Research, VISN 20 MIRECC (Mental Illness Research, Education and Clinical Center), and Chief, Psychiatric Research/ Psychopharmacology, Portland VA Medical Center; Professor of Psychiatry and Neurology, Oregon Health and Science University, Portland, Oregon

Carl I. Cohen, M.D.

Professor and Director, Division of Geriatric Psychiatry, Department of Geriatric Psychiatry, State University of New York Downstate Medical Center at Brooklyn, Brooklyn, New York

Francine Cournos, M.D.

Professor of Clinical Psychiatry, Columbia University College of Physicians and Surgeons; Director, Washington Heights Community Service, New York State Psychiatric Institute, New York, New York

Elissa Powers Ettinger, M.D.

Fellow in Psychiatry, Massachusetts General Hospital, Harvard Medical School, Boston, Massachusetts

Tony P. George, M.D.

Assistant Professor of Psychiatry, Yale University School of Medicine; Director, Dual Diagnosis and Smoking Research Program, Connecticut Mental Health Center and Substance Abuse Center, New Haven, Connecticut

Thomas E. Hansen, M.D.
Co-Manager, Acute Psychiatry, Portland VA Medical Center; Associate
Professor of Psychiatry, Oregon Health and Science University, Portland,
Oregon

David C. Henderson, M.D.
Associate Director, Psychotic Disorders and Schizophrenia Research Program, Massachusetts General Hospital; Assistant Professor of Psychiatry,
Harvard Medical School, Boston, Massachusetts

William G. Honer, M.D., F.R.C.P.C.
Professor, Department of Psychiatry, University of British Columbia,
Vancouver, British Columbia, Canada

Lili C. Kopala, M.D., F.R.C.P.C.
Director, Early Psychosis Program, and Professor, Department of Psychiatry, Dalhousie University, Halifax, Nova Scotia, Canada

Theo C. Manschreck, M.D., M.P.H.
Chief, Laboratory for Clinical and Experimental Psychopathology, and
Medical Director, John C. Corrigan Mental Health Center, VA Brockton
Psychiatry Services; Professor, Department of Psychiatry, Harvard Medical School, Fall River, Massachusetts

Karen McKinnon, M.A.
Research Scientist, New York State Psychiatric Institute; Project Director,
Columbia University HIV Mental Health Training Project, Columbia
University College of Physicians and Surgeons, New York, New York

Jonathan M. Meyer, M.D.
Assistant Professor of Psychiatry, Department of Psychiatry, University of
California, San Diego; Staff Psychiatrist, San Diego VA Medical Center,
San Diego, California

Henry A. Nasrallah, M.D.
Professor of Psychiatry, Neurology, and Neuroscience and Associate
Dean, University of Cincinnati College of Medicine, Cincinnati, Ohio

Alison Netski, M.D.
Resident Physician, University of Maryland Department of Psychiatry,
Baltimore, Maryland

Diana O. Perkins, M.D., M.P.H.
Associate Professor, Department of Psychiatry, University of North Carolina, Chapel Hill, North Carolina

Raymelle Schoos, M.D.
Resident Physician, State University of New York Downstate Medical Center at Brooklyn, Brooklyn, New York

Angelo Termine, B.S.
Research Associate, Program for Research in Smokers with Mental Illness, Connecticut Mental Health Center, and Yale University School of Medicine, New Haven, Connecticut

Jennifer C. Vessicchio, M.S.W.
Research Coordinator, Program for Research in Smokers with Mental Illness, Connecticut Mental Health Center, and Yale University School of Medicine, New Haven, Connecticut

Milton L. Wainberg, M.D.
Assistant Clinical Professor of Psychiatry, Columbia University College of Physicians and Surgeons, and Director of Medical Education, Columbia University HIV Mental Health Training Project, Columbia University College of Physicians and Surgeons; Adjunct Assistant Professor of Psychiatry, Mount Sinai School of Medicine, New York, New York

Christopher Welsh, M.D.
Assistant Professor of Psychiatry, University of Maryland Department of Psychiatry, Baltimore, Maryland

Donna A. Wirshing, M.D.
Associate Professor of Psychiatry, University of California, Los Angeles; and Chief, Schizophrenia Treatment Unit, West Los Angeles VA Medical Center, Los Angeles, California

Preface

The creation of this volume emerged out of the editors' recognition that there is a dearth of books on the subject of medical illness in schizophrenia, despite a growing body of literature. A *MEDLINE* search reveals that in 2001 there were 3,199 articles published that included the term *schizophrenia* or *antipsychotic*, of which 118 (3.69%) referred to weight gain or obesity, compared with 1,827 and 6 (0.33%) articles, respectively, in 1991. The increasing focus on medical morbidity and mortality among those with schizophrenia represents one aspect of a movement to extend the care of these patients beyond the treatment of psychotic symptoms, on the basis of empirical data linking medical comorbidity to overall outcomes. The literature of the last 5 years has increasingly demonstrated the need for more comprehensive medical assessment in patients with schizophrenia, because quality of life and indices of psychopathology are both adversely affected by the burden of medical illness (Dixon et al. 1999; Lyketsos et al. 2002). These findings are especially relevant in light of the fact that patients with schizophrenia suffer from increased rates of multiple medical problems due to lifestyle choices (e.g., high smoking prevalence, high-fat diet), effects of medications (e.g., obesity and diabetes mellitus related to certain atypical antipsychotics), inherent neglect of personal care, and barriers to treatment of physical illness (Cradock-O'Leary et al. 2002; Fontaine et al. 2001; Osby et al. 2000).

The chapters in this volume have been selected for their significant clinical relevance to the care of patients with severe mental illness. Those who publish in this area or manage patients with schizophrenia realize that psychiatrists have largely become the de facto primary care providers for these individuals. For all who maintain an academic or clinical interest in outcomes among schizophrenia patients, there is a tremendous need for a specialized volume that comprehensively addresses this important aspect of the overall care for these patients and that unifies the scattered published data on medical disorders overrepresented in this population. Although unnatural causes of death such as suicide and accidents account for a significant proportion of the mortality in this illness, cardiovascular causes alone may represent 50% or more of the excess mortality in schizophrenia. Given the likelihood that some of this medical burden (e.g., obesity, hyperlipidemia, diabetes mellitus) is iatrogenically induced by the use of certain antipsychotic medications (Meyer 2002; Nasrallah and Smeltzer 2002), it is incumbent on psychiatric physicians to take the lead in the monitoring of basic health care parameters. This is especially important for more occult but serious diseases such as human immunodeficiency virus (HIV) and hepatitis C, which are nearly 10 times more prevalent among the severely mentally ill than in the general population (Davidson et al. 2001).

The mind–body dualism that dominated psychiatric thinking for many decades has been transformed to a more holistic and integrated conceptualization of schizophrenia as a psychiatric disorder with neural underpinnings, for which findings from basic science and clinical research are utilized to generate new treatments. Because community mental health centers have become the focus not only for psychiatric care but also for vocational and social rehabilitation programs, a strong argument can be made—and runs as an underlying theme throughout this book—that the somatic needs of this vulnerable population must be actively addressed and not neglected in this setting. Awareness of the medical morbidities commonly seen in schizophrenia is a vital step toward both intervention in the disease process and advocacy for greater access to necessary services for this medically underserved population.

References

Cradock-O'Leary J, Young AS, Yano EM, et al: Use of general medical services by VA patients with psychiatric disorders. Psychiatr Serv 53:874–878, 2002

Davidson S, Judd F, Jolley D, et al: Risk factors for HIV/AIDS and hepatitis C among the chronic mentally ill. Aust N Z J Psychiatry 35:203–209, 2001

Dixon L, Postrado L, Delahanty J, et al: The association of medical comorbidity in schizophrenia with poor physical and mental health. J Nerv Ment Dis 187:496–502, 1999

Fontaine KR, Heo M, Harrigan EP, et al: Estimating the consequences of antipsychotic-induced weight gain on health and mortality rate. Psychiatry Res 101:277–288, 2001

Lyketsos CG, Dunn G, Kaminsky MJ, et al: Medical comorbidity in psychiatric inpatients: relation to clinical outcomes and hospital length of stay. Psychosomatics 43:24–30, 2002

Meyer JM: A retrospective comparison of lipid, glucose and weight changes at one year between olanzapine and risperidone treated inpatients. J Clin Psychiatry 63:425–433, 2002

Nasrallah HA, Smeltzer DJ: Contemporary Diagnosis and Management of the Patient With Schizophrenia. Newtown, PA, Handbooks in Health Care, 2002

Osby U, Correia N, Brandt L, et al: Mortality and causes of death in schizophrenia in Stockholm County, Sweden. Schizophr Res 45:21–28, 2000

Chapter 1

Issues Surrounding Medical Care for Individuals With Schizophrenia

The Challenge of Dual Neglect by Patients and the System

Jonathan M. Meyer, M.D.
Henry A. Nasrallah, M.D.

Introduction

The focus of schizophrenia research and treatment has broadened in the past decade beyond the narrow emphasis on positive and negative symptoms, which characterized the earlier approach to this disorder (Tsuang and Faraone 1999). Schizophrenia is now fully recognized as a multidimensional illness, with a profound impact on behavior, perceptions, thinking, emotions, neurocognition, and psychosocial functioning, that may not be fully managed with pharmacotherapy (O'Leary et al. 2000). The advent of rehabilitative models and multidisciplinary teams composed of mental health practitioners other than medical professionals has become the standard of care in many communities. This approach to schizophrenia treatment is centered on the need to remediate all aspects of dysfunction to maximize quality of life. Nevertheless, despite these efforts to provide more comprehensive services for the chronically mentally ill, data continue to demonstrate the substantial burden of medical comorbidity and excess mortality exacted from patients with schizophrenia (Brown et al. 2000). To be afflicted with schizophrenia implies a life expectancy approximately 20% shorter than that of the general population (Newman and Bland 1991), with much of this excess mortality due to medical causes rather than accidents or suicide, both of which are also prevalent. Many patients with schizophrenia receive little or no routine or preventive medical care during their interactions with the health care system in the United States, resulting in greater severity of illness and a higher burden of untreated medical conditions (Druss et al. 2002; Jeste et al. 1996). Although the focal point of contact for those suffering from schizophrenia is the psychiatric office or clinic, data from the National Ambulatory Medical Care Survey amassed from 1992 to 1999 on 3,198 office visits found that psychiatrists provided clinical preventive medical services in any form (e.g., health behavior and lifestyle counseling, measurement of blood pressure) to patients with severe mental illness during only 11% of visits (Daumit et al. 2002).

For many reasons, including the unfortunate dissociation of psychiatric and medical care that is common in the United States, and inherent aspects of the disorder, such as self-neglect, the medical needs of patients with schizophrenia often go unattended during the lifetime course of their psychiatric care (Stroup and Morrissey 2001). It should therefore not be surprising that patients with schizophrenia present with more advanced medical illness than do sex- and age-matched peers (Muck-Jorgensen et al. 2000), and that natural causes account for approximately half of the excess deaths in this population (Osby et al. 2000). This neglect and "myopia" regarding medical illness in schizophrenia care is not confined to community mental health practitioners, but is also reflected in the messages received from academia. Most textbooks on schizophrenia treatment devote little or no space to medical issues in this population, and typically offer no discussion about important sources of increased morbidity, including infectious diseases such as human immunodeficiency virus and hepatitis C, and cardiovascular disease, a primary source of excess mortality for these patients. The net result is not only shortened survival and decreased quality of life for those with schizophrenia due to the burden of untreated medical conditions, but also functional impairment and a direct adverse impact on psychiatric symptoms.

Two recent studies underscore this interaction between medical comorbidity and psychiatric status among patients with schizophrenia. That patient self-report about past medical service use is reliable in this population has been documented over the past decade, most recently in data demonstrating strong consistency among responses in a sample of 29 patients with schizophrenia who were interviewed two times, one week apart, regarding medical contacts over the past year (Goldberg et al. 2002). The survey interview method was employed by Dixon and colleagues to study a group of 719 patients with schizophrenia in various community settings as part of a Patient Outcomes Research Team (PORT) project examining the association between physical health, psychiatric symptoms, and quality of life (Dixon et al. 1999). After controlling for social and demographic factors, the authors concluded, "A greater number of current medical problems independently contributed to worse perceived physical health status, more severe psychosis and depression, and greater likelihood of a history of a suicide attempt (p. 496)."

Another study examined the association between physical health and psychiatric symptoms prospectively among 950 psychiatric admissions to the Johns Hopkins Hospital Phipps Psychiatric Service, of which 15.6% were diagnosed with schizophrenia. In those patients who received general medical health ratings, medical comorbidity was a focus of concern in 20% and represented a serious active problem in 15% at time of presentation; moreover, medical comorbidity was associated with a 10%–15% increase in psychiatric symptoms and functional impairment, controlling for clinical status at time of admission (Lyketsos et al. 2002).

Contributors to Medical Morbidity in Schizophrenia

Although these chapters illustrate the undeniable reality of excessive medical comorbidity in patients with schizophrenia, they also reflect a resurgent interest within the psychiatric community in defining the underlying systemic and illness-specific causes for this phenomenon, as evidenced in the growing body of literature on medical illness and health behaviors among the chronically mentally ill population.

Ranking high among the causes of poor physical health in schizophrenic patients are the unhealthy lifestyle practices so prevalent in this disorder. The fact that 70%–80% of patients with schizophrenia are chronic smokers has been extensively documented (Davidson et al. 2001), and studies of individuals with schizophrenia living in the community have also found a high prevalence of sedentary habits and poor dietary choices (Brown et al. 1999; Davidson et al. 2001). Comorbid substance use disorders have been shown to be common among patients with schizophrenia, and further contribute to poor physical health, less frequent medical follow-up, and an increased number and severity of medical conditions (Druss et al. 2002; Jeste et al. 1996).

Beyond lifestyle patterns, other factors associated with the diagnosis of schizophrenia appear to impede utilization of necessary medical services. Whether because of disorganization, negative symptoms, or the cognitive dysfunction associated with schizophrenia, multiple studies demonstrate that these individuals tend to have more limited contact with general medical professionals compared with other psychiatric and medical patients, even within systems of care such as the Veterans Affairs (VA) clinics, which facilitate access to primary care services. An extensive database review of 175,653 patients within the VA health care network in Southern California and Nevada seen during fiscal year 2000 found not only that the diagnosis of schizophrenia was highly correlated ($P < 0.001$) with fewer medical visits, but that fully two-thirds of those with schizophrenia had not even one diagnosis listed in their medical records among the highly prevalent diseases of the VA population: hypertension, diabetes mellitus, and chronic obstructive pulmonary disease (Cradock-O'Leary et al. 2002). A separate examination of medical or surgical follow-up care after psychiatric hospitalization in a national sample of veterans with comorbid medical disorders discharged from VA psychiatric units ($n = 44,533$) found that the diagnosis of schizophrenia was associated with a 31% reduced likelihood (odds ratio 0.69, 95% confidence interval [CI] 0.58–0.80) of an appointment within 30 days postdischarge (Druss and Rosenheck 1997). Moreover, those with schizophrenia took an average of 7.89 days longer to have the first medical visit, were 12% less likely to have any medical visit in the first 6 months after a follow-up appointment (odds ratio 0.88, 95% CI 0.79–0.97), and averaged 41% fewer visits during the 6 months after discharge. This study controlled for multiple variables, including proximity to the VA medical center, extent of patient VA financial support, and even proportion of individual hospital spending on medical and surgical services.

Once patients do establish contact with medical services, communication barriers may interfere with the provision of appropriate care. One 2-year prospective study noted that 24 of 28 patients with schizophrenia assessed at the end of the study were unable to name at least one of their physical problems (Pary and Barton 1988). It is reasonable to postulate that this communication difficulty may be the result of the cognitive dysfunction associated with schizophrenia, and such limitations in verbal expression combined with idiosyncratic, odd, or bizarre behavior certainly color interactions with nonpsychiatric medical professionals.

There are ample data suggesting that, overall, the quality of preventive care received by patients with schizophrenia is inferior to that of other groups, including those with other mental disorders. Druss and colleagues studied a database comprising 88,241 Medicare patients age 65 years and older hospitalized with clinically confirmed acute myocardial infarction (MI) to examine the quality of follow-up care for persons with mental disorders (Druss et al. 2001a). In their model comparing patients with specific psychiatric disorders with the rest of the population, patients with schizophrenia had a 34% increased risk of mortality in the year after hospital discharge for acute MI, whereas those with affective disorders had only an 11% increase. After the model was adjusted for quality measures and the covariates employed in the previous model, the association between mental disorders and 1-year mortality was no longer significant ($P=0.17$), implying that inadequate provision of standard quality measures after MI accounted for a substantial portion of the excess mortality experienced by post-MI patients with mental disorders. In particular, the excess mortality seen in schizophrenia became nonsignificant after adjustment for the provision of five quality measures: reperfusion therapy, aspirin, angiotensin-converting enzyme inhibitors, beta-adrenergic blockers, and counseling about smoking cessation (Druss et al. 2001a). In another large-database study of acute MI patients, those with schizophrenia were only 41% as likely to undergo cardiac catheterization as those without mental disorders ($P<0.001$) (Druss et al. 2000). Even female patients with schizophrenia who receive physical examinations or Pap smears at rates comparable to age-matched peers have surprisingly lower rates of mammography than the general population (62% vs. 86%), again implying unevenness in quality of care (Dickerson et al. 2002).

Another important contributor to adverse health outcomes is the side-effect profile of antipsychotic medications themselves. Numerous studies and reviews covered extensively later in this volume comment on the problems of obesity, hyperlipidemia, and type II diabetes mellitus in patients with schizophrenia exposed to certain atypical antipsychotics (Meyer 2001). This burden is added to what appears to be an underlying propensity in this population toward overweight and obesity, and greater prevalence of type II diabetes (Allison et al. 1999a, 1999b; Dixon et al. 2000). Nevertheless, as clinical researchers argue for the necessity of medical monitoring in patients receiving certain atypical antipsychotics, one fortuitous outcome is a renewed interest among mental health practitioners in means to integrate basic medical care into psychiatric practice, particularly in community mental health clinics (Meyer 2002).

Systems of Care

In the United States the community mental health center is the typical setting for providing chronically mentally ill patients with a panoply of interventions, including psychotropic medications, social work, and rehabilitative services (Lehman and Steinwachs 1998). Yet the near absence of preventive medical services in the psychiatric setting within the United States was confirmed by data from the National Ambulatory Medical Care Survey (Daumit et al. 2002), reflecting a mental health system "remarkable for its relatively high expenditures, for its fragmented services, and for its isolation from other medical fields" (Stroup and Morrissey 2001, p. 321). Since the mid-1950s both the United States and the United Kingdom have largely deinstitutionalized the care of patients with schizophrenia; yet treatment patterns in the UK stand in contrast to the prevalent community pattern in the United States of state or acute psychiatric hospital admissions followed by community mental health center psychiatric care, without a primary care link for the physical health of the patients. In the UK, general practitioners are the most commonly used service providers for the severely mentally ill, seen by 55% of patients with schizophrenia, whereas only 44% of this population receive care through psychiatric specialty clinics associated with hospitals (Stroup and Morrissey 2001). The fragmentation of health care in the United States reflects systemic issues that affect delivery in all fields of medicine but have an especially profound impact on medically vulnerable patients with schizophrenia, resulting in perpetuation of self-neglect, lack of early detection for medical illness, and potentially serious adverse effects of some medications.

Although the prospect of effecting change in the United States health care delivery systems engenders a certain amount of nihilism, a realistic approach to improving health for patients with schizophrenia must be determined by utilizing data from research initiatives (Le Fevre 2001). Only after careful assessment of feasibility, cost-effectiveness, and outcomes should certain approaches be abandoned. To specifically assess the impact of integrating medical and psychiatric care, investigators at the VA Healthcare System in West Haven, Connecticut, performed a 12-month prospective randomized study examining health delivery and outcomes for two groups of patients with serious mental disorders: those who received medical care as usual through the general medical clinics ($n=61$) and those assigned to an integrated psychiatric and medical clinic ($n=59$) (Druss et al. 2001b). Patients with schizophrenia made up 22.0% of the integrated-care group and 19.7% of the usual-care cohort. The primary source of medical care in the integrated model was a nurse practitioner who operated under the supervision of a family practitioner; additional nurse case manager and administrative support, to schedule appointments and telephone patients the day prior, was also provided in the integrated clinic. In particular, the integrated clinic staff made efforts to track and reschedule patients who missed appointments or failed to follow through with necessary care (e.g., laboratory testing). Outcome measures included total health care costs, quality of preventive care, satisfaction with medical care, physical health status as rated by the Short Form Health Survey (SF-36, a 36-item questionnaire with good reliability and consistency in this population), and mental symptoms according to the Symptom Checklist-90.

Quality and service utilization data were available for all patients at the end of 12 months, and survey data for 41 of 61 usual-care patients and 42 of 59 integrated-care patients, which reflect nearly identical rates of attrition for the two cohorts. Although the outcome measures were not broken down by diagnosis, the results are noteworthy nonetheless. Although total health care costs remained the same for the two groups despite the added personnel for the integrated clinic, integrated-care patients were significantly more likely to have a primary care visit in the year of observation than the usual-care group (91.5% vs. 72.1%; $P=0.006$) and significantly less likely to have an emergency department visit over the year (11.9% vs. 26.2%; $P=0.04$). The integrated-care group were also more likely to have received 15 of the 17 recommended preventive health measures, had markedly fewer problems regarding continuity of care compared with the usual-care sample (1.3% vs. 22.5%; $P<0.001$), and were significantly improved in ratings of physical health on the SF-36.

Although there are unique aspects of the VA health care system that may limit the generalizability of this model to community mental health centers (CMHCs), the fact that total health care costs did not increase bodes well for budget-strapped local governmental entities that staff and fund CMHCs. Clearly, the extension of such research to a patient population composed exclusively of those with schizophrenia receiving care in non-VA community clinics is needed to determine which aspects of this delivery model are feasible and effective in the CMHC setting.

Another option initially studied within the VA system is the use of a primary care psychiatrist to treat most common health conditions seen in the ambulatory care setting (Golomb et al. 2000). Such physicians would be psychiatrists with additional primary care training, supervised by an internist, who provide a level of care not obtainable through the use of non–psychiatrically trained medical personnel that may have difficulty establishing rapport with severely mentally ill patients or negotiating the interaction between fluctuations in psychiatric and medical symptoms. To determine which medical conditions would be appropriately treated by a primary care psychiatrist, a panel was convened among the chiefs of staff and representatives from psychiatry, internal medicine, and nursing services of three Southern California VA health care systems (West Los Angeles, San Diego, and Loma Linda) to assess the appropriateness of a primary care psychiatrist or more specialized medical intervention for 344 health conditions, procedures, and preventive care measures (Golomb et al. 2000). The basis for rating was a 10-point scale developed jointly by Rand and the University of California–Los Angeles (Brook et al. 1986), and ratings were performed by 11 physician members of the panel. Panel consensus at a rater agreement level of 7 out of 11 or higher determined primary care psychiatrists to be appropriate primary care providers for the majority of preventive screening and treatment items, for the majority of items related to evaluation and treatment of common medical conditions, and for common medical procedures. Consensus was especially high (85%) regarding the appropriateness of primary care psychiatrists for treatment of 11 of 13 conditions included in this study that rank among the top 20 most common reasons reported by patients for ambulatory care visits. Certainly the appeal of this model rests in the idea that persons seen by a primary care psychiatrist in a CMHC setting will receive integrated care in the form of a more medically oriented psychiatrist, thereby ensuring high levels of continuity and comfort with the care provider. Once again, the cost associated with the additional educational requirements, and the administrative feasibility of providing combined care in a CMHC (e.g., the format of supervision, requirements for new equipment and staffing), signal the need for further study.

Other tenable options include the dual training of physicians as board-certified psychiatrists and primary care physicians who can function independently without the need for supervision from an internist. Foreseeing the need for such dually trained physicians, the University of California–San Diego and the University of California–Davis have implemented combined training programs. These physicians could function as part of comprehensive health care teams, ideally situated within CMHCs, whose sole focus is the provision of integrated psychiatric and medical care to chronically mentally ill clients. Another model derives from an extension of the case management concept employed in most CMHCs to oversee integrated psychiatric and social care for patients. The West Haven VA study used a medical case manager as part of the intervention, whose major purpose was to ensure that patients kept appointments and that necessary testing was performed. Although integration of medical and psychiatric care within the CMHC may be ideal, in settings where administrative barriers prevent the implementation of this model, a medical case manager may be assigned to clients with identified health conditions to facilitate communication between psychiatric and medical care providers and to coordinate care.

Conclusion

In a special article published in the *American Journal of Psychiatry*, Lieberman and Rush (1996) discussed the changing roles psychiatrists must play in their approach to patient treatment in reaction to social, economic, and medical issues that define the parameters of care. They argued for the necessary reintegration of psychiatry within the specialties of medicine to prevent marginalization and to avoid perpetuation of the mind–body dichotomy that ultimately leads to compartmentalized care for patients such as those with schizophrenia, who typically possess multiple medical needs that are inadequately addressed in fragmented systems of care.

As will be described in the later chapters of this book, these medical needs in the schizophrenic population are daunting and unique. High rates of obesity, diabetes, substance use disorders, smoking, poor diet, sedentary lifestyle, and other unhealthy practices (such as unprotected sex, which increases the risk of infectious diseases such as human immunodeficiency virus and hepatitis C) combine with the negative symptoms and cognitive deficits associated with chronic psychosis to create significant barriers to health care access and a large reservoir of unmet medical needs (Dixon et al. 2001). Changes in health care policy and funding to facilitate the integration of medical service within the CMHC setting, and the increased availability of physicians trained as primary care psychiatrists, may effectively bridge the gap in access to and quality of medical care for the chronically mentally ill at some future date. In the meantime, psychiatrists and other psychiatric care providers cannot abjure their role as health care practitioners for this medically vulnerable population of individuals with chronic severe mental illness. An increased awareness of, and attention to, the basic monitoring requirements for common health conditions encountered among these patients may yield substantial reductions in morbidity and mortality, along with improvements in quality of life and reductions in level of functional impairment and psychopathology.

The overarching purpose of this volume is to serve as a useful reference about common medical conditions that should be a focus of clinical concern for those who encounter patients with schizophrenia, and thereby fill a long-standing need previously neglected in many practice settings and in the literature of disease management in schizophrenia. However, the implicit message underlying the creation of this book is that integration of medical and psychiatric care should be the norm, not the exception, and that psychiatrists must be in the forefront of advocacy for improved medical care for their patients with schizophrenia.

References

Allison DB, Fontaine KR, Heo M, et al: The distribution of body mass index among individuals with and without schizophrenia. J Clin Psychiatry 60:215–220, 1999a

Allison DB, Mentore JL, Heo M, et al: Antipsychotic-induced weight gain: a comprehensive research synthesis. Am J Psychiatry 156:1686–1696, 1999b

Brook RH, Chassin MR, Fink A, et al: A method for the detailed assessment of the appropriateness of medical technologies. Int J Technol Assess Health Care 2:53–63, 1986

Brown S, Birtwistle J, Roe L, et al: The unhealthy lifestyle of people with schizophrenia. Psychol Med 29:697–701, 1999

Brown S, Inskip H, Barraclough B: Causes of the excess mortality of schizophrenia. Br J Psychiatry 177:212–217, 2000

Cradock-O'Leary J, Young AS, Yano EM, et al: Use of general medical services by VA patients with psychiatric disorders. Psychiatr Serv 53:874–878, 2002

Daumit GL, Crum RM, Guallar E, et al: Receipt of preventive medical services at psychiatric visits by patients with severe mental illness. Psychiatr Serv 53:884–887, 2002

Davidson S, Judd F, Jolley D, et al: Cardiovascular risk factors for people with mental illness. Aust N Z J Psychiatry 35:196–202, 2001

Dickerson FB, Pater A, Origoni AE: Health behaviors and health status of older women with schizophrenia. Psychiatr Serv 53:882–884, 2002

Dixon L, Postrado L, Delahanty J, et al: The association of medical comorbidity in schizophrenia with poor physical and mental health. J Nerv Ment Dis 187:496–502, 1999

Dixon L, Weiden P, Delahanty J, et al: Prevalence and correlates of diabetes in national schizophrenia samples. Schizophr Bull 26:903–912, 2000

Dixon L, Wohlheiter K, Thompson D: Medical management of persons with schizophrenia, in Comprehensive Care of Schizophrenia: A Textbook of Clinical Management. Edited by Lieberman JA, Murray RM. London, Martin Dunitz, 2001, pp 281–292

Druss BG, Rosenheck RA: Use of medical services by veterans with mental disorders. Psychosomatics 38:451–458, 1997

Druss BG, Bradford DW, Rosenheck RA, et al: Mental disorders and use of cardiovascular procedures after myocardial infarction. JAMA 283:506–511, 2000

Druss BG, Bradford WD, Rosenheck RA, et al: Quality of medical care and excess mortality in older patients with mental disorders. Arch Gen Psychiatry 58:565–72, 2001a

Druss BG, Rohrbaugh RM, Levinson CM, et al: Integrated medical care for patients with serious psychiatric illness: a randomized trial. Arch Gen Psychiatry 58:861–868, 2001b

Druss BG, Rosenheck RA, Desai MM, et al: Quality of preventive medical care for patients with mental disorders. Med Care 40:129–136, 2002

Goldberg RW, Seybolt DC, Lehman A: Reliable self-report of health service use by individuals with serious mental illness. Psychiatr Serv 53:879–881, 2002

Golomb BA, Pyne JM, Wright, B et al: The role of psychiatrists in primary care of patients with severe mental illness. Psychiatr Serv 51:766–773, 2000

Jeste DV, Gladsjo JA, Lindamer LA, et al: Medical comorbidity in schizophrenia. Schizophr Bull 22:413–430, 1996

Le Fevre PD: Improving the physical health of patients with schizophrenia: therapeutic nihilism or realism? Scott Med J 46:11–13, 2001

Lehman AF, Steinwachs DM: Translating research into practice: the Schizophrenia Patient Outcomes Research Team (PORT) treatment recommendations. Schizophr Bull 24:1–10, 1998

Lieberman JA, Rush AJ: Redefining the role of psychiatry in medicine. Am J Psychiatry 153:1388–1397, 1996

Lyketsos CG, Dunn G, Kaminsky MJ, et al: Medical comorbidity in psychiatric inpatients: relation to clinical outcomes and hospital length of stay. Psychosomatics 43:24–30, 2002

Meyer JM: Effects of atypical antipsychotics on weight and serum lipids. J Clin Psychiatry 62 (suppl 27):27–34, 2001

Meyer JM: A retrospective comparison of lipid, glucose and weight changes at one year between olanzapine and risperidone treated inpatients. J Clin Psychiatry 63:425–433, 2002

Muck-Jorgensen P, Mors O, Mortensen PB, et al: The schizophrenic patient in the somatic hospital. Acta Psychiatr Scand Suppl 102:96–99, 2000

Newman SC, Bland RC: Mortality in a cohort of patients with schizophrenia: a record linkage study. Can J Psychiatry 36:239–245, 1991

O'Leary DS, Flaum M, Kesler ML, et al: Cognitive correlates of the negative, disorganized, and psychotic symptom dimensions of schizophrenia. J Neuropsychiatry Clin Neurosci 12:4–15, 2000

Osby U, Correia N, Brandt L, et al: Mortality and causes of death in schizophrenia in Stockholm County, Sweden. Schizophr Res 45:21–28, 2000

Pary RJ, Barton SN: Communication difficulty of patients with schizophrenia and physical illness. South Med J 81:489–490, 1988

Stroup TS, Morrissey JP: Systems of care for persons with schizophrenia in different countries, in Comprehensive Care of Schizophrenia: A Textbook of Clinical Management. Edited by Lieberman JA, Murray RM. London, Martin Dunitz, 2001, pp 315–326

Tsuang MT, Faraone SV: The concept of target features in schizophrenia research. Acta Psychiatr Scand Suppl 395:2–11, 1999

Chapter 2

Excessive Mortality and Morbidity Associated With Schizophrenia

Daniel E. Casey, M.D.
Thomas E. Hansen, M.D.

Introduction

Psychiatric conditions have long been recognized as carrying premature mortality. In his review, Brown (1997) noted that "lunatics" (perhaps 25% having schizophrenia) in a study from 1841 experienced mortality at between 3 and 14 times the rate seen in the general population. According to Brown, Eugen Bleuler reported that mortality in patients with schizophrenia was 1.4 times the expected rate, caused by food refusal, accidents, suicide, and infectious and other diseases from poor sanitation. Brown stated that although Kraepelin felt mortality was only slightly increased in dementia praecox, he still reported that suicide, negativism, diet, and poor cooperation with medical care contributed to increased mortality. Early modern data come from studies of mental hospitals and reflect the hazards of institutional care as well as contributions from the underlying psychiatric condition (Black et al. 1985; Brown 1997; Sims 2001). Brown (1997) reported that the standardized mortality ratio (SMR) found in studies from the first half of this century ranged between 210 and 400 (meaning mortality was between two and four times higher than expected in age- and gender-matched people from the general population). Mortality from tuberculosis and gastrointestinal infections was common in reports from earlier periods (Sims 2001), whereas unnatural causes (suicide and accidental death) became an increasingly important cause of premature death with the shift from inpatient to outpatient care for patients with schizophrenia (Black et al. 1985; Sims 2001). Cardiovascular disease and diabetes may be increasing in importance as causes of death and morbidity in more recent times (Jeste et al. 1996). With increasing concern about the metabolic consequences (weight gain, hyperglycemia, hyperlipidemia) of medications used to treat schizophrenia, a review of mortality and morbidity in schizophrenic patients, from natural as well as unnatural causes, should be useful to clinicians.

In this chapter, we review mortality rate data demonstrating that the life span for patients with schizophrenia is shortened. Many conditions that lead to premature death are evident during the patient's lifetime and account for the majority of the excess morbidity seen in schizophrenia. The disorders that do not necessarily lead to death but adversely affect patients with schizophrenia are discussed, along with patient and societal aspects of schizophrenia that might lead to poor health care.

Life Span and Mortality in Patients With Schizophrenia

Mortality Rates

Reviews of mortality rates in schizophrenia consistently find increased death rates in patients with schizophrenia. Reports commonly use record linkage methodology: databases of all deaths in a region are linked with population registers of psychiatric patients (community or hospital derived) so that the number of deaths in a group of patients with a specific diagnosis can be determined. This observed number is contrasted with the number expected based on life expectancy data for people of the same age and gender applied to the time period studied. The ratio of observed to expected cases is the SMR (some authors multiply the ratio by 100). In this chapter, we report the actual SMR figures used by authors, noting when the figure has been multiplied by 100. The 95% confidence interval (CI) values indicate statistical significance, with lower-CI values above 1.0 (or 100, when the SMR is multiplied by 100) supporting significance for elevated SMR, and upper-CI values below 1.0 (or 100) supporting significance for decreased SMR (Harris and Barraclough 1998). The consistent finding of higher rates is remarkable when one considers the variation in methods in both individual studies and reviews. For instance, individual studies from earlier periods may be overly influenced by inclusion of hospitalized patients (lower risk of suicide, higher risk of diseases related to institutionalization), and later studies are likely to include outpatients (greater risk of suicide) and to be more precise in diagnosis.

Three reviews that summarized results from studies conducted between 1942 and 1996 found the mortality rate in patients with schizophrenia to be between 1.5 and 2 times that expected. Allebeck (1989) reviewed nine studies published between 1942 and 1985 in which patients had been followed at least 5 years and he found mortality of about twice the expected rate. He noted difficulty in ascertaining whether rates had changed because diagnostic and study criteria had varied over time. Brown (1997) searched for studies published between 1986 and 1996 with schizophrenic patient populations of at least 100 individuals recruited after 1952 that included observed and expected death rates and had follow-up periods of at least 2 years, with losses to follow-up of less than 15%. He found an aggregate SMR of 151 (SMR × 100, 95% CI 148–154). The SMR for suicide was elevated at 838 (SMR × 100, 95% CI 784–894), as were the SMR for accidents (216, 95% CI 196–236) and the SMR for natural causes of death (110, 95% CI 105–115). He interpreted data about specific natural causes of death conservatively, stating that patients with schizophrenia die from the same diseases as the rest of the population. He did note that peptic ulcer (perhaps related to alcohol use) and pneumonia (probably associated with elderly institutionalized patients) caused death at higher-than-expected rates. Harris and Barraclough (1998) reviewed mortality rates in cohorts of patients with various mental disorders between 1966 and 1995 (20 studies, nine countries, almost 36,000 patients) and found a death risk in schizophrenic patients that was 1.6 times that expected. The mortality risk from unnatural causes (suicide and violence), 4.3 times that expected, exceeded the risk from natural causes (1.4 times that expected), but natural causes still accounted for 68% of the excess in expected deaths. Large individual studies may have influenced some of the authors' findings.

A number of studies published subsequent to these reviews are briefly reviewed here. Data from Stockholm County were included in the Allebeck review (1989); a subsequent nonoverlapping study from the same region (Osby et al. 2000a) followed mortality in 7,784 patients discharged from a first hospitalization for schizophrenia between 1973 and 1995. Data, reported by gender, reveal increased SMR for patients with schizophrenia (male 2.8, 95% CI 2.6–3.0; female 2.4, 95% CI 2.2–2.5). In an additional analysis (Osby et al. 2000b) of SMR by 5-year period of discharge, SMR increased significantly in more recent times, rising from 2.6 to 9.4 in males, and rising from 2.1 to 3.6 in females; the increase in relative risk of death was analyzed with multivariate regression models and found to be significant at $P=0.01$ for males and $P=0.05$ for females.

Two other recent studies also found higher mortality rates than in the older reviews. A cohort of 370 Southampton, England, outpatients with a diagnosis of schizophrenia treated during a 1-year period between 1981 and 1982 were followed for 13 years (Brown et al. 2000). The 79 patients who died led to an overall SMR ($\times$ 100) of 298 (CI 236–372). The authors suggested that this figure underestimates the actual impact of schizophrenia on mortality, because the age distribution of the population (middle-aged) means that included patients had already avoided a period of high risk for suicide, as discussed later. In a Finnish study (Joukamaa et al. 2001), 99 patients over 30 years of age, all having probable schizophrenia during 1977 to 1980, were identified, and mortality between 1978 and 1994 (15 to 17 years) was determined. (This was part of a larger study of other conditions.) The authors used a regression model to determine relative risk (RR) for death and found patients with schizophrenia to be at elevated risk (RR 3.29, 95% CI 2.21–4.91 for males; RR 2.26, 95% CI 1.33–3.84 for females).

Survival curve data offer a complementary approach that also finds increased mortality in patients with schizophrenia. For instance, in a Canadian study (included in the reviews noted earlier) of 3,623 patients treated during the 10-year period between 1976 and 1985, with an average follow-up interval of 6 years, 301 patients died (Newman and Bland 1991). SMR was 2.6. The authors determined, using survival curve analysis, that 85% of patients with schizophrenia would survive 10 years compared with an expected rate of 94%. They estimated life expectancy from birth of male patients to be only 56.2 years with schizophrenia compared with 72 years for the overall population in Alberta, and 66.1 years for females with schizophrenia compared with 79.1 years. Similarly, in a follow-up study of patients admitted to the University of Iowa Psychiatric Hospital between 1934 and 1944, 195 patients with schizophrenia were tracked and 60% were deceased as of 1974. Survival curve analysis revealed survival time shortened by 9 to 10 years. Finally, a recent Swedish study provided data on life expectancy in psychiatric conditions, including schizophrenia (Hannerz et al. 2001). The authors reported life expectancy by age group during 1983 for patients admitted to psychiatry clinics between 1978 and 1982. Life expectancies were calculated for patients and for the general population using actuarial mathematics. Schizophrenic patients had lower life expectancy, with the difference decreasing with increasing age. For instance, the decrease in life expectancy for 30-year-olds with schizophrenia in 1983 was 7.9 years for men and 9.5 years for women. Sixty-year-olds with schizophrenia in 1983 had decreases of 4.3 years for men and 3.2 years for women. The authors concluded that potential biases—the fact that patients had to have survived for 1 year after screening to be included favored longer survival, and the fact that patients were screened shortly after hospitalization meant that they were in a relatively intense phase of illness, favoring shorter survival—offset each other.

Examining sudden-death cases also demonstrates the increase in mortality associated with schizophrenia. All cases examined by the coroner's office in Victoria, Australia, during 1995 were cross-referenced with the psychiatric register (Ruschena et al. 1998). Patients on the psychiatric register were overrepresented in the sudden-death population; patients with schizophrenia had an RR of 4.9 (95% CI 4.1–5.9) in this study. Suicide was a common cause of death (50 out of 123 deaths in patients with schizophrenia), affecting younger patients commonly within 1 year of psychiatric hospitalization. An excess of death by natural causes was also seen in patients with schizophrenia (RR 2.9, 95% CI 2.1–3.9); cardiovascular disease accounted for the excess. Patients with schizophrenia were overrepresented in the "undetermined cause of death" group as well (RR 29.7, 95% CI 7.9–82.3).

Thus, data from the past 50 years demonstrate that the increase in mortality seen for patients with schizophrenia in earlier time periods persists. Furthermore, the disparity in death rates between patients with schizophrenia and the general population appears to be widening. Much additional information exists about the causes of this excess mortality.

Suicide and Other Unnatural Causes of Mortality

Reviews consistently find that suicide accounts for some of the increased mortality seen in patients with schizophrenia (Allebeck 1989; Harris and Barraclough 1998). This increased rate of death by suicide is evident in specific studies as well. In a 10-year follow-up of 1,190 patients with schizophrenia discharged from any hospital in Stockholm County in 1971 (Allebeck 1989; Allebeck and Wistedt 1986), 33 deaths out of 231 (14.3%) were registered as suicides, for an SMR of 12.3 (95% CI 9.1–15.6). Some accidental and undetermined deaths were probably suicides, so the actual rate was probably higher. In a subsequent study of a different patient group from Stockholm County (Osby et al. 2000a), 380 of 1,849 deaths (20.6%) were by suicide. The SMR for suicide deaths was 15.7 (95% CI 13.6–17.9) for males and 19.7 (95% CI 16.8–22.9) for females. The suicide

SMR was expected to be higher because this incidence study started following patients earlier in their illness, when suicide rates are higher. The authors also noted that the SMR for suicide in patients with schizophrenia appeared to be increasing. When the data were examined by 5-year period of admission (Osby et al. 2000b), the SMR for suicide in males went from 13.2 (1976–1980) to 47.8 (1991–1995), $P=0.07$, and in females from 17.1 (1976–1980) to 58.6 (1991–1995), $P=0.04$. One might expect the SMR for suicide to increase in later admission epochs, because the shorter follow-up period would include a proportionately larger amount of time with the patients at higher risk. However, that factor seems unlikely to explain this greater-than-threefold increase in SMR from suicide. The authors speculate that the patients admitted most recently have more severe illness (admission criteria being more stringent) but receive less intense care (despite more admissions, bed days of care fell, with a shift to more outpatient treatment).

These studies and several others are summarized in Table 2–1. The data support several observations. The increase in risk from suicide for patients with schizophrenia was much lower many years ago when patients were commonly kept in hospitals for long time periods (Mortensen and Juel 1990). The risk is greatest early in the course of illness and close to hospital discharge, so that mortality rates vary between studies depending in part on study inclusion criteria (Baxter and Appleby 1999; Brown and Birthwhistle 1996; Fenton 2000; Joukamaa et al. 2001). Finally, the risk of suicide appears to be increasing, perhaps related to greater reliance on less intensive treatment emphasizing outpatient care (Allebeck 1989; Osby et al. 2000a, 2000b).

To investigate concerns that psychiatric patients have a high death rate from unnatural deaths other than suicide, data on cause of death from accidents, homicides, and suicides were examined for 257,720 people admitted to Danish hospitals for psychiatric disorders between 1973 and 1993 (Hiroeh et al. 2001). The SMR ($\times$ 100) for male and female patients with a diagnosis of schizophrenia was elevated for suicide (males 1,073, 95% CI 973–1,183; females 1,080, 95% CI 936–1,246) and accidents (males 213, 95% CI 168–269; females 287, 95% CI 224–369). The absolute number of homicides was low (2 for women, 7 for men); the SMR was elevated for males (734, 95% CI 350–1,539) but not significantly so for females (341, 95% CI 85–1,363).

A national psychological autopsy study from Finland provided important details about the nature of suicide in patients with schizophrenia (Heila et al. 1997). All suicides occurring during a 1-year period during 1987 and 1988 were identified. Providers and next of kin were interviewed, and adequacy of medication was examined. This sample had a somewhat older age of suicide (mean 40 years) than hospital- or initially

Table 2–1. Mortality from suicide in patients with schizophrenia

Study	Period of follow-up	Mortality (SMR or other measure)	Deaths by suicide (% of all deaths)	Comment
Allebeck 1989	1971–1981	12.3 (95% CI 9.1–15.6)	14.3	
Osby et al. 2000a	1973–1995	15.7 male (95% CI 13.6–17.9), 19.7 female (95% CI 16.8–2.9)	20.6	Same area as Allebeck, more recent period
Brown et al. 2000	1981–1994	2,794 (×100) (95% CI 1,528–4,689)	33	
Newman and Bland 1991	1976–1985	19.6 ($P<0.04$)	33	Survival curve study
Joukamaa et al. 2001	1978–1994	12.4 (95% CI 2.81–54.7)	5.1	No female suicides Patients over 30 years old, survived 1 year before follow-up
Mortensen and Juel 1990	1957–1986	1.32 ($P<0.05$)	1.2	Most patients elderly, institutionalized
Fenton 2000	See comment	(6.4% of patients died by suicide)	43	Patients treated 1950–1975, additional follow-up unclear
Baxter and Appleby 1999	1969–1985	14.2 male (95% CI 9.2–x) 14.6 female (95% CI 8.8–x)	All cases suicides	Upper limit of CI not stated

Note.   SMR=standardized mortality ratio; 95% CI=95% confidence interval.

treated patient groups. The mean illness duration was 15.5 years, and 75% of patients had active symptoms. About 9% had current suicide command hallucinations. Twenty-five (27%) were hospitalized at the time of suicide, and 29 (32%) had been discharged within 3 months. A depressive syndrome had been present during either a residual or an active phase of psychosis in 61 patients (66%), with depressive symptoms at the time of suicide in 59 (64%). Drug overdose was the most common single cause of death (34 patients, 37%), although various violent means were used in 37 cases (40%). Of 34 drug overdoses, 27 (79%) were with neuroleptic medication and 25 (74%) specifically involved low-potency neuroleptics. The authors suspected that with the shift toward outpatient management, the availability of drugs to use in overdoses has increased. Additional data on risk factors and adequacy of treatment were reviewed for the 88 patients who were in treatment at the time of suicide (Heila et al. 1999). Data on compliance and treatment responsiveness were available for 72 patients. For the entire group of patients who committed suicide (either with active psychotic symptoms or during a residual phase of illness), only 34 (47%) appeared to be compliant and to be receiving an adequate dose of antipsychotic medication. Data were similar when the patients in active phase of illness were examined separately. Only 26 (46%) of the 57 patients experiencing active symptoms at the time of suicide were receiving an adequate dose (defined as 700 mg daily in chlorpromazine equivalents) and were compliant in taking medication. Other patients were noncompliant (17 of 57, 30%) or nonresponsive (14 of 57, 24%). Recently discharged patients (compared with inpatients or more remotely discharged patients) had the highest rates of alcohol abuse (36%), paranoid illness subtype (57%), and recent suicidality (74%). This group also had the highest number of lifetime hospitalizations per year of treatment (median of 1 compared with 0.43 and 0.27 for the other groups), with the shortest duration of recent hospitalization (median 24 days compared with 62 and 51.5 days in the other groups). Inclusion of these data suggests possible alternative interventions but cannot be conclusive because actual rates of suicide in groups are not known. These two studies suggest the importance of effective medication management and provision of appropriate intensity of treatment (if not inpatient, then close outpatient observation) in this era of managed care.

The data reviewed clearly demonstrate the importance of suicide in the increased mortality seen in patients with schizophrenia. Emphasis on SMR data may be misleading in terms of absolute risk, because suicide is rare and natural causes of death are far more common in the general population. As summarized in Table 2–1, roughly two-thirds of deaths in patients with schizophrenia are by causes other than suicide. Several alternative approaches to the data are instructive. For instance, the lifetime risk of suicide, defined as the proportion of all deaths contributed by suicide, addresses this issue. Data from a large meta-analysis (Harris and Barraclough 1998) were analyzed by plotting the percentage of patients who had died against the percentage of patients who died by suicide. The curve that best modeled the data was extrapolated to the point at which all members of the cohort would be deceased; the percentage of deaths by suicide out of all deaths was estimated to be 4%, lower than the frequently cited value of 10% lifetime risk for suicide in schizophrenia (Inskip et al. 1998). The proportion of excess deaths attributed to suicide also demonstrated that although many patients with schizophrenia die from suicide, far more die from other causes. As noted earlier, in the review done by Harris and Barraclough (1998), suicide accounted for 38% of the excess mortality. Consistent with this, in Brown's review (1997), 35% of excess mortality could be attributed to suicide, and in the cohort treated in 1981–1982 with 13 years of follow-up from Southampton, England, suicide and other unnatural causes accounted for 33% of the deaths (Brown et al. 2000). Another recent report (Osby et al. 2000a) found 24% of the excess deaths were from suicide. Another way to understand this issue is to note that although the relative risk for suicide in patients with schizophrenia compared with the general population is higher than the relative risk for natural causes of death, the absolute risk for natural causes of death is far higher than for suicide in patients with schizophrenia. Thus, excess mortality in schizophrenia derives primarily from natural causes rather than from suicide.

Natural Causes of Death in Patients With Schizophrenia

An autopsy study from the time when phenothiazine medications were new, roughly 50 years ago, provided a view of death by natural causes (Hussar 1966). Autopsy data from 1,275 chronically hospitalized patients with schizophrenia in a Veterans Affairs (VA) hospital who died at age 40 or older found that heart disease and cancer were the most common causes of death (similar to findings in the general 40+ population of that time). Pneumonia was somewhat overrepresented as a cause of death. Undetermined causes and aspiration of food were among the top eight causes of death in the patients with schizophrenia but not in the general population. The authors speculated that phenothiazines could be responsible, although they noted that other investigators at the time found no association between the new medications and death rates.

Harris and Barraclough (1998) reviewed mortality rates in cohorts of patients with various mental disorders between 1966 and 1995. Cohorts of patients with schizophrenia had an SMR (× 100) of 137 for natural causes, with significant increases in expected deaths from a variety of medical conditions (infectious, endocrine, circulatory, respiratory, digestive, and genitourinary disorders). Several subsequent studies have found a somewhat higher SMR for death by natural causes, with values of 232 (× 100, 95% CI 176–300) in one report (Brown et al. 2000), and 2.0 in males and 1.9 in females (95% CI 1.8–2.2 for males, and 1.8–2.0 for females) in another (Osby et al. 2000a). In a separate analysis of their data, the latter authors found that the SMR related to natural causes of death increased when rates were determined by 5-year periods (males increasing from 1.7 in 1976–1980 to 4.4 in 1991–1995, $P=0.02$; females showing an increase from 1.7 to 2.1 over the same interval, $P=0.04$) (Osby et al. 2000b).

Reviewing individual studies for increased risk of specific disorders is somewhat problematic. Many studies report categories of diseases from the *International Classification of Diseases* (ICD) rather than specific disorders. Also, findings vary between studies, perhaps because the SMR will be greatly influenced by a small number of observed cases when the expected rate is low. Given that reviews of studies, some including institutionalized patients, will present increased risks of certain diseases (infectious diseases, for instance), examining individual studies may be helpful in understanding risks for more recent periods. The failure to demonstrate increased risk of cancer when all causes of cancer are aggregated has led to much speculation. The persistence and increase in both deaths from and risk for disorders such as cardiovascular disease and diabetes is also important.

When all types of cancer are included, mortality for patients with schizophrenia ranges from very similar to nonsignificantly elevated over expected. Specific results include SMR of 100 (× 100, meaning that the number observed was the same as the number expected) (Harris and Barraclough 1998), 1.1 (Newman and Bland 1991), 1.1 for males and 1.3 for females (Osby et al. 2000a), 1.46 (Brown et al. 2000), and 1.4 (Allebeck 1989). A decreased rate of lung cancer in males has been noted to offset increases in other types of cancer, such as breast cancer in females (Mortensen and Juel 1990) or digestive cancers (Newman and Bland 1991). In the latter study, the SMR for lung cancer was 0.7 (not significantly decreased) and for digestive cancer was 1.7 ($P<0.05$). Limited access to cigarettes for institutionalized patients has been raised as a possible explanation for reduced rates of lung cancer (Harris and Barraclough 1998).

To investigate the reported decrease in mortality from lung cancer, Masterson and O'Shea (1984) looked at rates of smoking in 100 chronic inpatients with schizophrenia in about 1984 and at cause of death in 122 patients who died in the same hospital between 1974 and 1983. The proportion of deaths from respiratory cancers was not significantly different from that for the general population (3.3% vs. 4.3%). The authors expected a higher rate of respiratory cancers in the patients with schizophrenia because the rate of smoking was higher in patients compared with the general public and because the rate of death from pneumonia (presumably linked to smoking) accounted for more deaths in patients with schizophrenia compared with the general population (18.8% vs. 6.5%, $P<0.001$). The authors speculated that the failure to see an increase in lung cancer deaths suggested antitumor activity by phenothiazine medication. However, an alternative explanation may be that patients die from other causes such as cardiovascular disease before they reach the expected age of death from lung cancer. Despite this possible antitumor activity, breast cancer caused proportionately more deaths in the schizophrenic patients (8.3% vs. 3.4% in the general population, $P<0.04$). The authors also speculated that being nulliparous and having elevated prolactin, both associated with schizophrenic illness and treatment, while practicing inadequate breast care (insufficient self-examinations and incomplete reporting of lumps) could have caused the increase in breast cancer.

Two incidence studies on cancer in patients with schizophrenia further demonstrate varying results between geographic locations for different types of cancer. The results varied between cohorts in the World Health Organization's three-cohort study (Gulbinat et al. 1992). The Danish cohort showed decreased rates of cancer (standardized incidence ratio [SIR] 0.67, 95% CI 0.60–0.75), the Nagasaki cohort revealed increased risk of cancer (male SIR 1.43, not significant, with 95% CI 0.85–2.26; female SIR 1.67, 95% CI 1.17–2.44), and the Honolulu cohort overall demonstrated no unusual cancer incidence (females of Japanese origin did have elevated risk, with an SIR of 1.73, 95% CI 1.03–2.74). Different patterns of risk were seen between cohorts when the data were analyzed by site of malignancy. The Danish group had low rates of lung, prostate, cervical, and ovarian cancers, whereas breast cancer was increased in the Nagasaki and Honolulu Japanese females and cervical cancer in the Nagasaki females. The authors concluded that patients with schizophrenia do not demonstrate any consistent increase or decrease in risk for cancer. In contrast, the authors of a records linkage study between the Finnish cancer and psychiatric illness registries found a modest but significantly elevated SIR for cancer (1.17, 95% CI 1.09–1.25) in patients with schizophrenia (Lichtermann et al. 2001), with the incidence of lung cancer twice as high in patients with schizophrenia (SIR 2.17, 95% CI 1.78–2.60). They also noted that the incidence of cancer of the gallbladder was elevated (SIR 2.07, 95% CI 1.03–3.70) and wondered about the role of obesity and poor diet in patients with schizophrenia, given that these are risk factors for gallstones, and hence possibly for gallbladder cancer. The authors did not find a significantly increased incidence of breast cancer (SIR 1.15, 95% CI 0.98–1.34) but did find a higher rate of uterine cancer (SIR 1.75, 95% CI 1.19–2.48), suggesting obesity, low levels of physical activity, and lower parity as possible causes. The inconsistency of these findings with the other cancer incidence and mortality studies in schizophrenia dictates caution in accepting these as correct. For instance, still another study suggests increased risk of breast cancer. Breast cancer was found at a higher rate on mammograms done for all female psychiatric patients at the Buffalo Psychiatric Center compared with women who had been referred for mammograms to the same radiology service because of possible breast disease (Halbreich et al. 1996). Thus, one cannot draw a firm conclusion about whether any type of cancer is increased or decreased in patients with schizophrenia.

On the other hand, many other diseases do clearly contribute to increased mortality in schizophrenia, including respiratory, endocrine, and cardiovascular diseases. In their review, Harris and Barraclough (1998) found an SMR for respiratory disease in patients with schizophrenia of 214 in males (95% CI 191–238) and 249 in females (95% CI 223–278). Subsequent studies confirm this rate, with an SMR of 317 (95% CI 116–690) in one (Brown et al. 2000); 9.5 in males (95% CI 3.8–23.8) and 8.3 in females (95% CI 2.58–26.84) in a second (Joukamaa et al. 2001); and 3.2 in males (95% CI 2.4–4.2) and 2.7 in females (95% CI 2.1–3.4) in a third (Osby et al. 2000a).

Although an elevated SMR for endocrine disorders was not reported in the review article (Harris and Barraclough 1998), several separate studies have found an increase in SMR. In one, the SMR was 2.7 for males (95% CI 1.6–4.2) and 2.0 for females (95% CI 1.1–3.4) (Osby et al. 2000a). In the other, the SMR for all endocrine disorders was 1,166 (× 100, 95% CI 379–2,721), with diabetes having an SMR of 996 (× 100, 95% CI 205–2,911) (Brown et al. 2000). A future increase in the SMR for diabetes might be anticipated, given the probable association between use of atypical antipsychotic medications and diabetes (Muench and Carey 2001).

Cardiovascular disease causes a large number of deaths in both the general population and patients with schizophrenia. In the review by Harris and Barraclough, circulatory diseases caused 2,313 deaths out of the 5,591 deaths from natural causes, leading to an SMR in males of 110 (× 100, 95% CI 104–116) and in females of 102 (× 100, not significant, 95% CI 96–108) (Harris and Barraclough 1998). Although the increase in risk is relatively small, the number of excess deaths is substantial (230 more than expected compared with a total of excess deaths from natural causes of 1,250). Subsequent studies found higher cardiovascular mortality rates. In one, circulatory disease had an SMR of 249 (× 100, 95% CI 164–363), and more specifically, cardiovascular disease had an SMR of 187 (95% CI 102–298) (Brown et al. 2000). Only males demonstrated an increase in relative risk for cardiovascular deaths in another study (RR 2.92, 95% CI 1.65–5.2). In a third, the SMR for cardiovascular disease was 2.3 for males (95% CI 2.0–2.6) and 2.1 in females (95% CI 1.9–2.4) (Osby et al. 2000a).

The increase in SMR from cardiovascular disease seen in these studies compared with older reports might reflect an important trend of increasing risk for patients with schizophrenia relative to the comparison group. The data in the last study reported above were reanalyzed by 5-year periods from 1976 to 1995 (Osby et al. 2000b). The SMR, reflecting mortality rates above those in comparable people from the general population, rose sharply, with the SMR for males increasing from 1.7 in 1976–1980 to 8.3 in 1991–1995 ($P < 0.001$) and for females from 1.7 to 5.0 over the same period ($P < 0.002$). If in fact risks of mortality from schizophrenia are increasing, then increased attention to the risks of cardiovascular disease in schizophrenia such as weight gain, smoking, hyperlipidemia, hypertension, and diabetes will be needed (Fontaine et al. 2001; Muench and Carey 2001). (For further information, please see other chapters in this volume: Chapter 3, "Obesity in Patients With Schizophrenia"; Chapter 4, "Cardiovascular Illness and Hyperlipidemia in Patients With Schizophrenia"; Chapter 5, "Nicotine and Tobacco Use in Schizophrenia"; and Chapter 6, "Glucose Intolerance and Diabetes in Schizophrenia.")

These data demonstrate that a number of medical conditions, especially cardiovascular disease and diabetes, contribute to the increased mortality related to natural causes seen in patients with schizophrenia. These diseases, and others, might also be expected to cause increased morbidity.

Morbidity in Schizophrenia

Medical Conditions

In reviewing several Danish reports on medical conditions in patients with schizophrenia, Munk-Jorgensen et al. (2000) found one study in which 70% of 399 acutely admitted psychiatric patients had medical problems (38% previously undiagnosed) and another in which 50% of 174 had somatic illnesses (31% previously undiagnosed). The authors also determined the rate ratio for various pulmonary and cardiovascular diseases in patients with schizophrenia identified through records linkage methodology. Most lung diseases but only some cardiovascular diseases had elevated rate ratio values. In a study of 110 state hospital patients with schizophrenia in the United States, 38 (35%) had one or more medical conditions (excluding extrapyramidal side effects and tardive dyskinesia) (Pary and Barton 1988). The disorders noted included diabetes, hyponatremia, thyroid disorder, urinary tract infection, bladder dysfunction, hypertension, liver disease, seizures, and visual problems, among others.

Similar rates of medical problems were found in a survey interview study of patients with schizophrenia from the Patient Outcomes Research Team program (Dixon et al. 1999). Of 719 patients, 469 (65%) reported having at least one lifetime medical condition, 256 (36%) had more than one condition, and 343 (48%) said the medical condition was active. The authors did not have a comparison control group but noted that the rates for diabetes, hypertension, and cardiac diseases were all higher than the rates reported for these conditions in the National Health Interview Survey. Not surprisingly, the number of medical comorbidities correlated significantly with patient self-rating of physical health.

Jeste et al. (1996) reviewed reports on medical comorbidity in schizophrenia; for unclear reasons, rheumatoid arthritis seems to occur only rarely in patients with schizophrenia, and cardiovascular disease and diabetes mellitus may be increased in patients with schizophrenia (although not unique to the illness, because affective disorders and other psychiatric illnesses may also be associated with increased risk). Consistent with the preceding review for mortality data, Jeste et al. (1996) reported that studies vary in finding increased rates of other specific illnesses and that the impression of decreased risk of cancer does not appear to be valid. The authors presented additional data from two morbidity studies of middle-aged to elderly patients with schizophrenia. In the first, patients with schizophrenia were contrasted with a group of patients with depression and with another group with Alzheimer's disease. They found lower rates of physical illnesses in the patients with schizophrenia. These data do not address whether medical illnesses are increased in schizophrenia versus the general population. In the second study, 45 patients with schizophrenia were compared with 38 normal control subjects; patients in both groups were 45 years of age or older. Indications of morbidity were comparable in the groups, but the control group was about 10 years older than the group of patients with schizophrenia. The authors also noted that patients with schizophrenia acknowledged more medical concerns when questioned in a structured manner.

Evaluating morbidity associated with schizophrenia is complicated by the lack of a uniform definition for morbidity, underreporting of physical illnesses by patients and medical providers, and the role of medications in causing some of the physical illnesses (Adler and Griffith 1991). One approach to these problems is to study hospitalizations for medical problems in patients with schizophrenia. For instance, the rates of medical hospitalizations and surgical procedures were determined for the population of patients who were identified with schizophrenia in Oxfordshire, England, between 1971 and 1973 (Herrman et al. 1983). Overall, the rate of general hospital discharges for patients with schizophrenia was elevated, but this was largely accounted for by hospitalizations for accidents, violence, and poisoning. The authors pointed out that the low rate of hospitalizations for other medical conditions may be a consequence of patients receiving treatment in psychiatry wards for medical problems. Also, the rate of surgical procedures was decreased (about 0.8) for schizophrenia patients. The authors speculated that physicians may have been reluctant to refer patients with schizophrenia for elective procedures.

The expected increase in morbidity was seen in a case-control study of hospitalizations in Stockholm (Dalmau et al. 1997). The authors gathered data for treatment of somatic conditions in 775 schizophrenic and 775 case-matched control subjects regardless of whether the treatment occurred in a psychiatric or a general medical ward. The schizophrenic group had 523 admissions (67%) compared with 373 (48%) for the control group over the 15-year study period (McNemar test, $P=0.000$). An increased odds ratio was found for almost all medical disorders occurring in patients with schizophrenia, with the exception of genitourinary, musculoskeletal, and sensory organ diseases. Tumors (combined malignant and benign) were found twice as often in schizophrenic patients.

In summary, the data demonstrate increased morbidity from medical conditions in patients with schizophrenia. Almost all disorders can occur at a higher-than-expected rate, particularly for cardiovascular disease and diabetes.

Substance Abuse

Patients with schizophrenia have increased rates of all types of substance abuse (Dixon 1999; Cantor-Graae et al. 2001; Swofford et al. 2000; Walkup et al. 2001), as covered in detail later in this text (Chapter 9, "Substance Use Disorders in Schizophrenia"). The adverse psychiatric effects (Dixon 1999; Swofford et al. 2000) combined with medical problems caused by substance abuse lead to the expectation of increased morbidity and mortality in patients with schizophrenia who abuse drugs or alcohol. Thus, Dalmau et al. (1997) found that inclusion of schizophrenic patients with substance abuse in their study cohort increased the number of somatic conditions that occurred more frequently in schizophrenic patients than in a nonpsychiatric control population.

Health Maintenance in Patients With Schizophrenia

Treatment Concerns

Treatment in the first half of the twentieth century undoubtedly contributed to morbidity and mortality in schizophrenia. Physical interventions such as leukotomy, insulin coma therapy, and cardiazol-induced convulsive therapy all carried substantial risk (Brown 1997). In the past 50 years, morbidity and mortality concerns related to treatment have shifted to medications. Several studies suggest the potential influence of antipsychotic medications on mortality in patients with schizophrenia. In an autopsy register study, the authors noted that 3 of the 10 cases in which no cause of death could be established despite a full autopsy had a diagnosis of schizophrenia (2 had other psychiatric diagnoses). This led to the question of whether medications could be responsible, although there was no evidence of antipsychotic medication levels outside the therapeutic range (Ruschena et al. 1998). Waddington et al. (1998) conducted a 10-year follow-up study of mortality and medication use in patients with schizophrenia. They found that antipsychotic polypharmacy and absence of co-treatment with anticholinergic medication significantly increased mortality. No clear explanation related to other factors that might co-vary with polypharmacy seemed plausible, leaving the authors to wonder whether concurrent use of multiple antipsychotic medications causes some adverse biological consequence, or whether unrecognized subclinical drug-induced parkinsonism could contribute to mortality. Certainly, extrapyramidal side effects, including tardive dyskinesia, cause substantial morbidity in patients with schizophrenia (Casey 1993; Hansen et al. 1997). Other chapters in this volume address neurological disorders (see Chapter 10, "Neurological Comorbidity and Features in Schizophrenia") and the contribution of atypical antipsychotic medications to various metabolic problems such as diabetes, hyperlipidemia, and obesity (see Chapter 3, "Obesity in Patients With Schizophrenia"; Chapter 4, "Cardiovascular Illness and Hyperlipidemia in Patients With Schizophrenia"; Chapter 5, "Nicotine and Tobacco Use in Schizophrenia"; and Chapter 6, "Glucose Intolerance and Diabetes in Schizophrenia").

Patient Health Habits and Related Concerns

Behaviors such as abuse of drugs and alcohol, smoking, lack of exercise, and dietary indiscretion appear to contribute to mortality in the general population, and thus are likely to do so in patients with schizophrenia (Brown et al. 1999). Brown et al. (2000) noted that the SMR related to natural causes of death was significantly ($P=0.05$) elevated in smokers (360 [× 100], 95% CI 270–471) but not in nonsmokers (178, 95% CI 85–328). The authors reviewed apparently avoidable natural causes of death in these patients. Causes included failure to recognize medical disease by the patient or care provider (three to eight cases), missed diagnoses (three cases), poor treatment compliance (unable to quantify), treatment refusal (two cases), and inadequate social support (one case).

Brown et al. (1999) directly investigated lifestyle concerns in 102 patients with schizophrenia. Patients with schizophrenia ate a diet significantly higher in fat and lower in fiber (significant for males, trend for females) compared with the reference population. Roughly one-third of the patients with schizophrenia reported doing no exercise, and no patient reported doing strenuous exercise (comparison rates not provided). In their sample, female patients demonstrated a trend toward obesity ($P=0.09$). The rate of smoking was higher in patients with schizophrenia (68% vs. 28% in males, 57% vs. 25% in females); alcohol consumption was decreased in males and unexceptional in females. A study of 22 outpatients with schizophrenia conducted in 1992–1993 found similar results (Holmberg and Kane 1999): patients with schizophrenia were less likely to practice health-promoting behaviors than nonpsychiatric populations. In a study of smoking in Irish inpatients with schizophrenia (Masterson and O'Shea 1984), the rate of smoking was higher than for the general population (males 84% vs. 41%, females 82% vs. 36%), as were daily consumption of cigarettes, preference for medium- to high-tar cigarettes (59% vs. 1%), and duration of smoking (longer than 16 years, 80% vs. 56%). The sum of the evidence indicates clearly that patients with schizophrenia engage in behaviors that can be expected to increase morbidity and mortality.

Access to Health Care

One can easily conjecture that decreased access to either medical or psychiatric care could exacerbate morbidity and contribute to increased mortality in patients with schizophrenia. For instance, in reporting increasing SMRs in Stockholm County for patients admitted during more recent 5-year periods, Osby et al. (2000b) point out that a shift from inpatient to outpatient care occurred. They suggest that the increase in SMR related to suicide and violence may be related to decreased intensity of care, with bed days of care declining despite increasing admissions of patients with more severe illnesses.

A number of reports suggest that access to medical care may be limited for patients with schizophrenia. Multiple factors could contribute to decreased access, including limitations in the communication of symptoms by patients, poor cooperation by psychotic patients, prejudice (based on fear, frustration, or anxiety) against schizophrenic patients, and insufficient attention to medical problems by mental health providers (Adler and Griffith 1991; Druss and Rosenheck 1997; Goldman 1999; Pary and Barton 1988). Dixon et al. (1999) found that less than 70% of the patients with medical problems were receiving treatment for their medical conditions in a survey interview study of 719 patients from the Patient Outcomes Research Team project. Masterson and O'Shea (1984) speculated that inadequate breast examinations and incomplete reporting of breast lumps could have contributed to the increased rate of death from breast cancer in their report. Herrman et al. (1983) suggest that bias against referring patients with schizophrenia for elective procedures could account for a decreased rate of surgeries in such patients in Oxfordshire, England. The diagnosis of schizophrenia was significantly negatively associated with timeliness, access, and intensity of postdischarge medical care in a study of United States veterans (Druss and Rosenheck 1997). Finally, two related studies have demonstrated disparity in care for patients with schizophrenia following myocardial infarction. Patients with schizophrenia ($n=188$) were less likely to have cardiac catheterization, more likely to die in the year after discharge, and less likely to receive interventions that represent quality of care following acute myocardial infarction—reperfusion therapy, aspirin, beta-blockers, and angiotensin-converting enzyme inhibitors (Druss et al. 2000, 2001).

Among the homeless, having a diagnosis of schizophrenia may be associated with better care and reduced mortality compared with the general homeless population. The age-adjusted mortality rate for a New York City homeless sample (follow-up period 1987–1994) was about four times that in a comparable reference group (Barrow et al. 1999). Having a mental illness had a significant protective effect, possibly explained by provision of more services and better housing for the homeless mentally ill compared with other homeless people. Likewise, having schizophrenia appeared to convey protection from mortality in a Boston homeless population (Hwang et al. 1998). The benefit of additional care most likely creates only an impression of protection, considering that the comparison groups are highly ill and impoverished. For example, mortality was studied in homeless individuals who had been referred to a clinic in Sydney, Australia, between 1988 and 1991 (Babidge et al. 2001). The SMR for the nonschizophrenic group was 4.41 (95% CI 2.02–6.19) compared with 2.52 (95% CI 1.8–3.43) for the schizophrenic group. Thus, although the SMR was much lower in the schizophrenic group, it still represented a mortality rate more than twice that expected in the general population.

Conclusion

The literature conclusively establishes that patients with schizophrenia die at higher rates and earlier than other people. The causes of this excess mortality have varied over time, reflecting issues related to changes in the care of patients with schizophrenia and the unhealthy lifestyles that result from a combination of their illness and the type of care available. At this time, interventions must address risks from suicide and from medical illnesses. Effective medications with side-effect profiles that promote adherence to treatment plans must be provided. Avoiding adverse metabolic side effects, or at least monitoring and attempting to correct them as they occur, is also critical in reversing the trend toward higher mortality in patients with schizophrenia. Finally, the mental health system must work to ensure that adequate social services, medical treatment, and psychiatric care are provided despite society's drive to reduce health care costs.

References

Adler LE, Griffith JM: Concurrent medical illness in the schizophrenic patient: epidemiology, diagnosis, and management. Schizophr Res 4:91–107, 1991

Allebeck P: Schizophrenia: a life-shortening disease. Schizophr Bull 15:81–89, 1989

Allebeck P, Wistedt B: Mortality in schizophrenia: a ten-year follow-up based on the Stockholm County inpatient register. Arch Gen Psychiatry 43:650–653, 1986

Babidge NC, Buhrich N, Butler T: Mortality among homeless people with schizophrenia in Sydney, Australia: a 10-year follow-up. Acta Psychiatr Scand 103:105–110, 2001

Barrow SM, Herman DB, Cordova P, et al: Mortality among homeless shelter residents in New York City. Am J Public Health 89:529–534, 1999

Baxter D, Appleby L: Case register study of suicide risk in mental disorders. Br J Psychiatry 175:322–326, 1999

Black DW, Warrack G, Winokur G: The Iowa record-linkage study, I: suicides and accidental deaths among psychiatric patients. Arch Gen Psychiatry 42:71–75, 1985

Brown AS, Birthwhistle J: Excess mortality of mental illness. Br J Psychiatry 169:383–384, 1996

Brown S: Excess mortality of schizophrenia: a meta-analysis. Br J Psychiatry 171:502–508, 1997

Brown S, Birtwistle J, Roe L, et al: The unhealthy lifestyle of people with schizophrenia. Psychol Med 29:697–701, 1999

Brown S, Inskip H, Barraclough B: Causes of the excess mortality of schizophrenia. Br J Psychiatry 177:212–217, 2000

Cantor-Graae E, Nordstrom LG, McNeil TF: Substance abuse in schizophrenia: a review of the literature and a study of correlates in Sweden. Schizophr Res 48:69–82, 2001

Casey DE: Neuroleptic-induced acute extrapyramidal syndromes and tardive dyskinesia. Psychiatr Clin North Am 16:589–610, 1993

Dalmau A, Bergman B, Brismar B: Somatic morbidity in schizophrenia: a case control study. Public Health 111:393–397, 1997

Dixon L: Dual diagnosis of substance abuse in schizophrenia: prevalence and impact on outcomes. Schizophr Res 35 (suppl):S93–S100, 1999

Dixon L, Postrado L, Delahanty J, et al: The association of medical comorbidity in schizophrenia with poor physical and mental health. J Nerv Ment Dis 187:496–502, 1999

Druss BG, Rosenheck RA: Use of medical services by veterans with mental disorders. Psychosomatics 38:451–458, 1997

Druss BG, Bradford DW, Rosenheck RA, et al: Mental disorders and use of cardiovascular procedures after myocardial infarction. JAMA 283:506–511, 2000

Druss BG, Bradford WD, Rosenheck RA, et al: Quality of medical care and excess mortality in older patients with mental disorders. Arch Gen Psychiatry 58:565–572, 2001

Fenton WS: Depression, suicide, and suicide prevention in schizophrenia. Suicide Life Threat Behav 30:34–49, 2000

Fontaine KR, Heo M, Harrigan EP, et al: Estimating the consequences of antipsychotic-induced weight gain on health and mortality rate. Psychiatry Res 101:277–288, 2001

Goldman LS: Medical illness in patients with schizophrenia. J Clin Psychiatry 60 (suppl 21):10–15, 1999

Gulbinat W, Dupont A, Jablensky A, et al: Cancer incidence of schizophrenic patients: results of record linkage studies in three countries. Br J Psychiatry Suppl 75–83, 1992

Halbreich U, Shen J, Panaro V: Are chronic psychiatric patients at increased risk for developing breast cancer? Am J Psychiatry 153:559–560, 1996

Hannerz H, Borga P, Borritz M: Life expectancies for individuals with psychiatric diagnoses. Public Health 115:328–337, 2001

Hansen TE, Casey DE, Hoffman WF: Neuroleptic intolerance. Schizophr Bull 23:567–582, 1997

Harris EC, Barraclough B: Excess mortality of mental disorder. Br J Psychiatry 173:11–53, 1998

Heila H, Isometsa ET, Henriksson MM, et al: Suicide and schizophrenia: a nation-wide psychological autopsy study on age- and sex-specific clinical characteristics of 92 suicide victims with schizophrenia. Am J Psychiatry 154:1235–1242, 1997

Heila H, Isometsa ET, Henriksson MM, et al: Suicide victims with schizophrenia in different treatment phases and adequacy of antipsychotic medication. J Clin Psychiatry 60:200–208, 1999

Herrman HE, Baldwin JA, Christie D: A record-linkage study of mortality and general hospital discharge in patients diagnosed as schizophrenic. Psychol Med 13:581–593, 1983

Hiroeh U, Appleby L, Mortensen PB, et al: Death by homicide, suicide, and other unnatural causes in people with mental illness: a population-based study. Lancet 358:2110–2112, 2001

Holmberg SK, Kane C: Health and self-care practices of persons with schizophrenia. Psychiatr Serv 50:827–829, 1999

Hussar AE: Leading causes of death in institutionalized chronic schizophrenic patients: a study of 1,275 autopsy protocols. J Nerv Ment Dis 142:45–57, 1966

Hwang SW, Lebow JM, Bierer MF, et al: Risk factors for death in homeless adults in Boston. Arch Intern Med 158:1454–1460, 1998

Inskip HM, Harris EC, Barraclough B: Lifetime risk of suicide for affective disorder, alcoholism and schizophrenia. Br J Psychiatry 172:35–37, 1998

Jeste DV, Gladsjo JA, Lindamer LA, et al: Medical comorbidity in schizophrenia. Schizophr Bull 22:413–430, 1996

Joukamaa M, Heliovaara M, Knekt P, et al: Mental disorders and cause-specific mortality. Br J Psychiatry 179:498–502, 2001

Lichtermann D, Ekelund J, Pukkala E, et al: Incidence of cancer among persons with schizophrenia and their relatives. Arch Gen Psychiatry 58:573–578, 2001

Masterson E, O'Shea B: Smoking and malignancy in schizophrenia. Br J Psychiatry 145:429–432, 1984

Mortensen PB, Juel K: Mortality and causes of death in schizophrenic patients in Denmark. Acta Psychiatr Scand 81:372–377, 1990

Muench J, Carey M: Diabetes mellitus associated with atypical antipsychotic medications: new case report and review of the literature. J Am Board Fam Pract 14:278–282, 2001

Munk-Jorgensen P, Mors O, Mortensen PB, et al: The schizophrenic patient in the somatic hospital. Acta Psychiatr Scand Suppl 102:96–99, 2000

Newman SC, Bland RC: Mortality in a cohort of patients with schizophrenia: a record linkage study. Can J Psychiatry 36:239–245, 1991

Osby U, Correia N, Brandt L, et al: Mortality and causes of death in schizophrenia in Stockholm County, Sweden. Schizophr Res 45:21–28, 2000a

Osby U, Correia N, Brandt L, et al: Time trends in schizophrenia mortality in Stockholm County, Sweden: cohort study. BMJ 321:483–484, 2000b

Pary RJ, Barton SN: Communication difficulty of patients with schizophrenia and physical illness. South Med J 81:489–490, 1988

Ruschena D, Mullen PE, Burgess P, et al: Sudden death in psychiatric patients. Br J Psychiatry 172:331–336, 1998

Sims AC: Mortality statistics in psychiatry. Br J Psychiatry 179:477–478, 2001

Swofford CD, Scheller-Gilkey G, Miller AH, et al: Double jeopardy: schizophrenia and substance use. Am J Drug Alcohol Abuse 26:343–353, 2000

Waddington JL, Youssef HA, Kinsella A: Mortality in schizophrenia: antipsychotic polypharmacy and absence of adjunctive anticholinergics over the course of a 10-year prospective study. Br J Psychiatry 173:325–329, 1998

Walkup JT, McAlpine DD, Olfson M, et al: Is the substance abuse of inpatients with schizophrenia overlooked? Gen Hosp Psychiatry 23:26–30, 2001

Chapter 3

Obesity in Patients With Schizophrenia

Donna A. Wirshing, M.D.
Jonathan M. Meyer, M.D.

The Epidemic of Obesity

Obesity and its related sequelae represent a growing epidemic in the United States. Overweight is defined by the World Health Organization as a body mass index (BMI) of 25.0–29.9 kg/m^2, and obesity as BMI $\geq$ 30 kg/m^2. Recent data estimate that more than 50% of U.S. adults are overweight, with 31% of men and 35% of women considered obese, or at least 20% above their ideal body weight (Yanovski and Yanovski 1999). Results of the 1999 National Health and Nutrition Examination Survey (NHANES), released in December 2000 by the National Center for Health Statistics, noted that the proportion of obese individuals in the United States in 1999 was 80% greater than the proportion measured by NHANES II in 1976–1980, and 17% greater than that measured by NHANES III in 1997 (Flegal and Troiano 2000). Similarly, the Centers for Disease Control (CDC) performed a telephone survey in 1991 that found that only 4 of the 47 states surveyed had obesity rates of 15% or greater, whereas the 2000 survey, which was repeated in all 50 states, found that every state except Colorado had an obesity rate $\geq$15% (Mokdad et al. 2000a, 2000b).

The economic burden of health care costs related to obesity has also grown dramatically in the past decade. Direct health costs of obesity in the United States were over $50 billion in 1995, or 7% of the total U.S. health care budget (Wolf and Colditz 1998), whereas both direct and indirect costs of obesity were estimated to be $98 billion in 1997 and $241 billion in 2001 (Schlosser 2001). This compares with an estimated $17.3 billion for direct health care costs of schizophrenia in the United States in 1995, with indirect costs of close to $50 billion (Knapp 2000). A major source of the health care costs for obesity relates to the development of comorbid medical disorders, particularly diabetes mellitus, which itself accounts for approximately 60% of the health care costs attributed to obesity (Colditz 1999). Other conditions such as hypertension, coronary heart disease, cholelithiasis, arthritis, and certain cancers (e.g., breast) become increasingly prevalent as BMI increases into the overweight and obese range (Must et al. 1999).

In addition to the health care costs of obesity, social stigma, discrimination, and low self-esteem are common problems among patients with obesity (Myers and Rosen 1999). This stigmatization can lead to psychological distress and could exacerbate illness in the vulnerable, psychotic individual. The stigma of mental illness combined with that of being overweight or obese is a significant burden for patients suffering from both conditions.

Obesity in Schizophrenia

In the pre-antipsychotic era, Kraepelin noted that some patients with schizophrenia exhibited bizarre eating habits, and not uncommonly were obese. "The taking of food fluctuates from complete refusal to the greatest voracity. The body weight usually falls at first often to a considerable degree.... [L]ater, on the contrary we see the weight not infrequently rise quickly in the most extraordinary way, so that the patients in a short time acquire an uncommonly well-nourished turgid appearance" (Kraepelin 1919, p. 125). It is worth noting that this tendency to weight loss during more active phases of the illness has been borne out by results from a recent meta-analysis of multiple antipsychotic drug trials, which noted that placebo-treated patients on average lost weight (Allison et al. 1999a). Nevertheless, there are a number of reasons that patients with schizophrenia might be prone to obesity, including the effect of symptoms such as paranoia and negative symptoms such as apathy and social withdrawal, which may independently contribute to schizophrenic patients' lack of adherence to proper diet and their overall sedentary lifestyle (Davidson et al.

2001). Moreover, the economic conditions of chronically mentally ill individuals also contribute to poor dietary habits. One theory about the major vector of the obesity epidemic in this country and abroad correlates obesity trends with the growth of the fast-food industry (Schlosser 2001). Fast food is an affordable option for those on limited budgets, yet unfortunately is often very high in saturated fat and total calories.

The Effects of Antipsychotic Medications on Weight

Antipsychotic medications have been the mainstay of treatment for schizophrenia for over half a century. A link between weight gain and treatment with chlorpromazine and other low-potency conventional antipsychotic agents, such as thioridazine, was noted in early studies of the metabolic effects of these agents. (Bernstein 1988; Rockwell et al. 1983). A recent study by Allison et al. (1999b) based on 1989 National Health Interview Survey data revealed that a significantly greater proportion of female patients with schizophrenia had BMI distributions in the overweight and obese spectrum compared with their counterparts in the general medical population, with a trend toward greater BMI seen among male schizophrenic patients. This study is notable because the data are based on survey material collected in 1989, before the advent of the novel antipsychotic medications. Thus, the results of that survey reflect obesity in a population of schizophrenic patients medicated with conventional antipsychotic medications. In general, treatment with lower-potency conventional antipsychotics was associated with greater weight gain than treatment with higher-potency agents. Over 10 weeks of treatment with conventional agents, mean gains of 2.65 kg were seen with chlorpromazine and 3.19 kg with thioridazine, compared with only 1.1 kg with the high-potency agent haloperidol (Allison et al. 1999a). The pharmacology of obesity will be discussed later in this chapter, but the greater propensity for histamine H_1 antagonism is thought to be the primary reason that lower-potency agents were associated with greater weight gain than higher-potency drugs such as haloperidol or fluphenazine.

Since the late 1980s a number of novel antipsychotic medications have been developed and released for clinical use worldwide. Unlike typical antipsychotics, the novel agents clozapine, risperidone, olanzapine, quetiapine, and ziprasidone are weaker dopamine D_2 antagonists, and therefore have very favorable extrapyramidal side-effect profiles compared with conventional antipsychotic agents. Unfortunately, some of the novel agents appear to have significant liabilities in terms of weight gain, especially compared with high-potency conventional drugs such as haloperidol. Wirshing and colleagues published a retrospective study of 122 clinical records of 92 outpatients involved in long-term clinical trials and found that clozapine therapy was associated with the most weight gain (6.9 ± 0.8 kg) among the novel antipsychotic medications examined (controlling for patient age and treatment duration), followed by olanzapine (6.8 ± 1.0 kg), risperidone (5.0 ± 0.6 kg), and the conventional agent haloperidol (3.7 ± 0.6 kg) (Wirshing et al. 1999). Allison and colleagues' comprehensive meta-analysis of 81 clinical trials with data on antipsychotic-induced weight gain (Allison et al. 1999a) found that the dibenzodiazepine-derived novel antipsychotics clozapine and olanzapine demonstrated weight gain at 10 weeks of therapy exceeding even that seen with thioridazine (clozapine 4.45 kg, olanzapine 4.15 kg); lesser gains were seen with risperidone (2.1 kg) and ziprasidone (0.04 kg). Ten-week data were not available for quetiapine.

Long-term data with clozapine- and olanzapine-treated patients also document weight gain far in excess of that seen with the low-potency typical antipsychotics such as chlorpromazine or thioridazine, whereas risperidone and ziprasidone show lower weight gain propensities, and conflicting data exist regarding quetiapine. Mean increases reported during the first year of therapy are 5.3–6.3 kg for clozapine and 6.8–11.8 kg for olanzapine, with substantial proportions in each group gaining more than 20% of their initial body weight in this time frame (Bustillo et al. 1996; Henderson et al. 2000; Kinon et al. 2001; Nemeroff 1997). Package insert information on olanzapine reports that over 50% of patients treated in long-term studies gained more than 7% of their initial body weight. Although risperidone and quetiapine have more weight gain propensity than that associated with a high-potency agent such as haloperidol, their reported mean gains of 2.0–2.3 kg and 2.77–5.60 kg, respectively, over 12 months compare favorably with clozapine, olanzapine, and low-potency typical antipsychotics (Jones et al. 2000; Marder 1997; Taylor and McAskill 2000); however, recent long-term data from Canada showed weight gain related to quetiapine therapy of 7.6 kg, much closer to that seen with olanzapine and clozapine (McIntyre et al. 2001). Interestingly, retrospective data published by Reinstein found that quetiapine, when added to patients' clozapine regimen after clozapine dose reduction, resulted in weight loss. However, it is difficult to know if co-treatment with quetiapine or the dosage reduction of clozapine was responsible for the weight loss observed (Reinstein et al. 1999). Ziprasidone was released in the United States in 2001, and long-term studies show a mean gain of 0.23 kg at 6 months, with 14.0% gaining ≥7% of their baseline weight at 10.5 months (Pfizer 2000).

The relative propensity for weight gain with atypical antipsychotic medications is reflected in the manufacturers' package inserts, which must include FDA-mandated data on the percentage of patients who gained ≥7% of their initial body weight during short-term premarketing clinical trials. The reported percentages are as follows: olanzapine 29%, quetiapine 23%, risperidone 18%, and ziprasidone 10% (Zyprexa 2000; Seroquel 2000; Risperdal 1999; Geodon 2001, respectively).

The time course in the progression of weight increase varies with the potential of each individual agent to cause weight gain. For those atypicals associated with greater weight gain, namely olanzapine and clozapine, a plateau appears between 39 and 52 weeks of therapy, although patients on clozapine may continue to gain approximately 4 pounds per year through the fourth year of treatment (Henderson et al. 2000; Kinon et al. 2001). In patients receiving ziprasidone, risperidone, or quetiapine, the plateau occurs much earlier, typically during the first few months of treatment (Brecher and Melvin 2001; Green et al. 2000; Taylor and McAskill 2000). Wirshing and colleagues also noted in their retrospective study that patients treated with clozapine and olanzapine had weight gain over longer periods of time compared with risperidone- and haloperidol-treated patients (Wirshing et al. 1999). They observed that patients gained weight over at least 20 weeks on clozapine and olanzapine, compared with approximately 10 weeks during treatment with risperidone.

The literature on weight gain with novel antipsychotic medications indicates that certain groups of patients, such as adolescents, may be particularly susceptible to this problem. In a retrospective study, Theisen and colleagues reported that the prevalence of obesity in adolescent patients was 64% on clozapine ($n=69$) and 56% on other atypicals (olanzapine, sulpiride, and risperidone) ($n=27$), compared with 30% for adolescent patients on conventional antipsychotic medications ($n=20$) and 28% for patients on no medications ($n=25$) (Theisen et al. 2001).

In an attempt to understand patient characteristics that may be predictors of weight gain on atypical antipsychotics, several retrospective studies have examined correlations between clinical response and weight gain. There are several conflicting reports about the relationship between weight gain and clinical improvement on atypical antipsychotic medications (Gupta et al. 1999; Leadbetter et al. 1992; Umbricht et al. 1994). Investigators from Eli Lilly, Inc., retrospectively analyzed their data from olanzapine trials and concluded that patients who were thinnest gained the most weight (Basson et al. 2001) and that there was a correlation between clinical improvement and weight gain. No relationship between either olanzapine dose or quetiapine dose and weight gain has been established (Brecher and Melvin 2001). Prospective research to determine which patient population or patient characteristics increase vulnerability to weight gain is still sorely needed.

Psychopharmacology of Weight Gain

Novel antipsychotic medications and conventional antipsychotic medications affect a number of central neurotransmitter systems that may have an impact on satiety and feeding behavior. Many of the receptor systems blocked by antipsychotic medications are those that are stimulated by medications that promote weight loss. For example, all antipsychotic medications block dopamine D_2 and noradrenergic α_1 receptors, the same sites stimulated by amphetamines and sympathomimetic amine drugs used to promote weight loss. Additionally, psychotropic drugs influence serotonin (5-HT) and histamine H_1 neurotransmission, both of which have been reported to affect food intake and cause fluctuations in weight.

In examining the binding profiles of antipsychotic agents, the receptor affinity characteristic most closely correlated with weight gain among novel antipsychotic medications was H_1 antagonism (Wirshing et al. 1999) (see Figure 3–1). Although H_1 blockade also causes sedation, the mechanism by which H_1 receptor antagonism may increase weight is peripheral interference with normal satiety signals from the gut, resulting in overeating (Knight 1985; Rockwell et al. 1983). Both low-potency conventional agents and those novel antipsychotic medications with higher weight gain potential have substantial affinity for this receptor (Schotte et al. 1993); however, what may contribute to the greater weight gain seen with some of the novel antipsychotics is the additional effect of $5\text{-}HT_{2C}$ antagonism.

Since the advent of clozapine, novel antipsychotics have been designed primarily to be both relatively weak D_2 antagonists and potent antagonists at $5\text{-}HT_{2A}$ receptors, yet these agents also have substantial affinity for the closely related $5\text{-}HT_{2C}$ receptor. It is known that compounds that stimulate 5-HT transmission reduce food consumption and cause weight loss (e.g., *m*-chlorphenylpiperazine, fenfluramine, sibutramine) whereas drugs that decrease 5-HT transmission increase food intake and are associated with weight gain (Goodall et al. 1988; Samanin and Garattini 1990). It is unclear which 5-HT receptor type is responsible for stimulating food intake and weight gain (Aulakh et al. 1992), but data implicate antagonism of $5\text{-}HT_{2C}$ receptors as a possible site where novel antipsychotics might have an impact on weight (Tecott et al. 1995). Evidence for this assertion comes from two types of data. Drugs such as fenfluramine are thought to suppress appetite via $5\text{-}HT_{2C}$ agonism (Garattini et al. 1989); moreover, Tecott and colleagues developed a strain of mice in which the gene coding for the

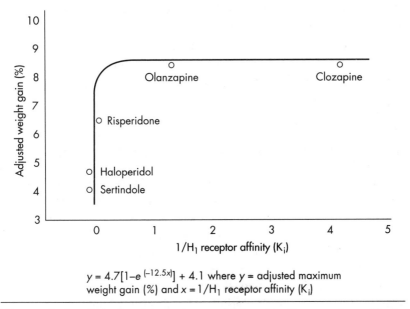

$$y = 4.7[1-e^{(-12.5x)}] + 4.1 \text{ where } y = \text{adjusted maximum}$$
weight gain (%) and $x = 1/H_1$ receptor affinity (K_i)

Figure 3–1. Relationship between histamine H_1 receptor affinity and adjusted weight gain among antipsychotics.

Source. Reprinted from Wirshing D, Wirshing W, Kysar L, et al.: "Novel Antipsychotics: Comparison of Weight Gain Liabilities." *Journal of Clinical Psychiatry* 60:358–363, 1999. Used with permission.

$5-HT_{2C}$ receptor was knocked out. As these mice age, they become obese, and also develop type II diabetes mellitus (Tecott et al. 1995). Although most of the novel antipsychotic medications are indeed $5-HT_{2C}$ antagonists, the propensity for weight gain best correlates not with the rank order of $5-HT_{2C}$ antagonism, but with the potency of histamine H_1 antagonism.

Another mechanism by which novel antipsychotics may have an impact on weight is via effects on peptide hormones. Leptin is a hormone produced by adipose tissue that is thought to signal the size of the pool of adiposity to the brain and thereby decrease feeding behavior. In humans, circulating leptin correlates closely with BMI (Kraus et al. 1999). Mice and humans deficient in leptin are obese, whereas parenteral administration of exogenous leptin reverses the abnormalities in food intake and weight in leptin-deficient individuals (Pelleymounter et al. 1995). An early paper examining clozapine-treated patients found increases in both adipose tissue and circulating levels of leptin (Bromel et al. 1998). In a subsequent study which found that leptin was increased in patients treated with clozapine or olanzapine but not with haloperidol, the investigators speculated that the normal hormonal feedback mechanism was impaired in patients taking those novel antipsychotic medications (i.e., they continue to overeat despite high circulating leptin levels) (Kraus et al. 1999). Moreover, an 8-week study found significant increases in body weight, serum leptin levels, and percentage of body fat in patients treated with olanzapine, but not in the drug-free comparison group (Eder et al. 2001).

Weight Monitoring for Schizophrenia

The effects of antipsychotic-related weight gain have both medical and psychiatric components. In particular, medication compliance is adversely affected by excessive weight gain, with weight gain being a well-known cause of treatment nonadherence (Bernstein 1988; Silverstone et al. 1988) and subsequent psychotic relapse (Rockwell et al. 1983). During the 2000 American Psychiatric Association meeting, investigators at the Columbia–St. Luke's Obesity Research Center released survey data examining this link between obesity and antipsychotic medication compliance. They found that obese patients were 13 times as likely to request discontinuation of their current antipsychotic agent because of concerns about weight gain and 3 times as likely to be noncompliant with treatment compared with nonobese individuals (Weiden et al. 2000). Patients who gain weight on antipsychotics also utilize health care resources more than patients who do not experience weight gain (Allison and Mackell 2000).

The first step in the battle against obesity and novel antipsychotic medication–associated weight gain is to appreciate the severity of this ubiquitous problem. Much as clinicians became aware of tardive dyskinesia as a long-term extrapyramidal side effect related to conventional antipsychotic therapy, there is increasing concern among mental health professionals about the long-term impact of weight gain. The initial choice of antipsychotic agent appears to play a significant role in the development of weight gain. Moreover, the concomitant use of other agents associated with weight gain, such as lithium or valproate, has been demonstrated to increase weight gain at 1 year to 16 pounds in risperidone-treated inpatients and over 27 pounds in olanzapine-treated inpatients (Meyer 2002). A new antipsychotic that came to the United States market in the last quarter of 2002, aripiprazole, looks promising in terms of its weight gain profile (Petrie et al. 1997), adding another medication to the armamentarium of novel antipsychotic agents with low propensity for weight gain.

In this age of second-generation antipsychotic medications, we need to routinely ask patients if they notice a change in their waist size or increased appetite, and intervene early, when weight gain is modest (i.e., 5 pounds).

Prevention in this case may be the greatest cure. Physicians should routinely measure weight at each visit, and BMI should be recorded. The National Heart, Lung and Blood Institute (NHLBI) has posted a useful, free BMI calculator for Palm operating system–based PDAs on its Web site (hin.nhlbi.nih.gov/bmi_palm.htm). An even more important predictor of diabetes and the dysmetabolic syndrome (also known as syndrome X, a quartet of symptoms including hypertriglyceridemia, diabetes, hypertension, and abdominal obesity) (Groop and Orho-Melander 2001) is waist circumference, a reflection of visceral adiposity (Park et al. 2001). Central adiposity is more highly associated with diabetes, the dysmetabolic syndrome, and subsequent increased risk of coronary artery disease. A waist circumference of ≥40 inches in males and ≥35 inches in females should prompt referral for more thorough health screening of lipids, glucose, and blood pressure. These combined medical consequences of obesity may thus offset to some extent the benefit gained from the antipsychotic agent's life-saving potential (Fontaine et al. 2001).

Patients with schizophrenia should be given nutritional counseling and recommendations for an exercise regimen, given their propensity for poor dietary habits and sedentary lifestyle. Primary care practitioners, family members, and other caregivers should be alerted to the risk of obesity during treatment with certain novel antipsychotics, as the potential complications of weight gain in patients with schizophrenia can be serious. It is also essential that patients be educated regarding the weight gain liability of their antipsychotic medication to minimize the risks of obesity and its related health consequences. Multiple cases of new-onset diabetes (Wirshing et al. 2001a), hyperlipidemia (Meyer 2001; Wirshing et al. 2001b), and sleep apnea have been reported as potentially associated with antipsychotic-related weight gain (Furst et al. 2002), although there may also be effects of certain novel antipsychotics on glucose tolerance and lipids independent of their effects on weight. (Monitoring recommendations for serum lipids and blood glucose are discussed in Chapter 4 and Chapter 6, respectively, in this volume.)

Behavioral Treatment

Behavioral interventions such as calorie restriction, exercise, and behavioral modification are key elements to successful, sustained weight loss (NHLBI 2000; NHLBI also has posted on its Web site a practical guide for obesity evaluation and management: www.nhlbi.nih.gov/guidelines/obesity/practgd_c.pdf). There is little in the way of published data on behavioral interventions for weight loss in psychotic patients, and the few studies tend to be methodologically weak. In one small $(n=14)$ 14-week study, patients in a residential setting achieved, on average, 10 pounds more weight loss when given behavioral interventions compared with a control group (Rotatori 1980). Work by Wirshing and colleagues demonstrated that simple stepwise behavioral interventions were modestly successful in risperidone- and olanzapine-treated subjects, but had little effect in clozapine-treated subjects (Wirshing et al. 1999). The interventions are listed below.

1. Patients were instructed to weigh themselves and report their weight to the clinic nurse at each visit (every 1–4 weeks).
2. If this simple behavioral intervention failed (a gain of 10 pounds was generally considered sufficient to warrant further intervention), patients were instructed to keep a detailed diary of all food intake over a several-week period; the diary was reviewed and recommendations made for changes in diet. If the food diary failed to maintain or decrease weight, patients were referred to a clinical nutritionist.
3. If the previous measures failed, individuals were sent to the Wellness Clinic at the medical center, which involved a more rigorous evaluation of both dietary and exercise habits and added education, exercise classes, and group support.

Although it is true that not all subjects availed themselves of these services, there is no reason to think that any one drug group would have more or fewer "noncooperative" patients. Final weight gains reported by Wirshing and colleagues for olanzapine and risperidone were 2.4 ± 1.3 kg and 2.3 ± 0.8 kg, respectively, compared with maximum weight gains achieved on these medications of 6.8 ± 1.0 kg (olanzapine) and 5.0 ± 0.6 kg (risperidone). In addition to this work, there have been reports suggesting that there may be some benefit to programs such as Weight Watchers in addressing novel antipsychotic–associated weight gain, although the dropout rate was quite high (10 of 21) in one recent study, and only the men experienced significant weight loss (Ball et al. 2001).

Pharmacological Treatment of Obesity in Schizophrenia

The literature thus far suggests that some of the novel antipsychotic medications cause less weight gain than others; thus it may be possible to switch patients on agents associated with the most weight gain to those with lower weight gain liability (Allison et al. 1999a; Wirshing et al. 1999); however, prior to switching, it is important to recall that the most difficult symptoms to control are those of psychosis. A switch of antipsychotic medication makes sense particularly if the patient is nonresponsive to the current antipsychotic. As discussed, weight gain can be a significant cause of nonadherence with a medication regimen; thus, in cases where a patient refuses to take medication due to weight gain concerns, a switch is advisable (Bernstein 1988; Silverstone et al. 1988). A switch study sponsored by Pfizer demonstrated that subjects switched from olanzapine to ziprasidone lost a statistically significant 2.2 kg on average over 6 weeks (Kingsbury et al. 2001). Moreover, recent preliminary data from a Janssen-sponsored study suggest improvements in both weight and markers of glucose tolerance in patients switched from olanzapine to risperidone (Berry and Mahmoud 2001). There is no current evidence that medications other than clozapine are highly effective in treatment-refractory patients, so caution must be exercised in deciding to switch a patient from clozapine.

There have been few studies involving the administration of weight loss agents to psychotic patients. The National Institutes of Health (NIH) guidelines allow the use of weight loss agents for patients with a BMI ≥ 27 kg/m^2 and obesity-related complications. Weight loss agents can also be administered to patients with BMI ≥ 30 kg/m^2 who do not have obesity-related complications (Aronne 2001). Amantadine, fenfluramine, and chlorphentermine have been used with moderate success (Correa et al. 1987; Kolokowska et al. 1987), although there are concerns that these drugs may worsen psychotic symptoms, and fenfluramine is no longer available on the market due to complications of cardiac valve dysfunction and pulmonary hypertension.

Medications that have been recently indicated for weight loss such as sibutramine and orlistat (Cerulli et al. 1998) have not been methodically tried or reported in this patient population. Sibutramine is a serotonin and norepinephrine reuptake inhibitor that was originally developed as an antidepressant, but was instead approved by the FDA as a treatment for obesity (Luque and Rey 1999). Orlistat is an inhibitor of gastric and pancreatic lipases that decreases dietary fat absorption, resulting in lowering of body weight and plasma cholesterol (Cerulli et al. 1998). Orlistat is difficult to administer, requiring three-times-daily dosing and fat-soluble vitamin supplementation, and thus may be difficult to use in psychiatric populations; however, because it does not have CNS effects it may be useful in this population (Hilgar et al. 2002).

Unapproved options for obesity treatment that may be of benefit include topiramate, histamine H$_2$ antagonists, and metformin. Topiramate, a new anticonvulsant that is being tested for its safety and efficacy in the treatment of bipolar disorder, causes a decrease in appetite and sustained weight loss in obese individuals. It has not been systematically studied as primarily a weight loss agent but has demonstrated weight loss in patients with epilepsy and bipolar disorders (McElroy et al. 2000; Norton et al. 1997; Rosenfeld et al. 1997) and is being tested in binge-eating disorder (Yanovski and Yanovski 2002). The use of H_2 antagonists for weight loss has been suggested in the literature, with speculation that H_2 antagonism may affect weight either by decreasing appetite via increases in cholecystokinin, a hormone that may signal satiety to the brain, or through the suppression of gastric acid secretion, which may decrease appetite (Sacchetti et al. 2000). Nizatidine, a histamine H_2 blocking agent, was recently compared with placebo as an adjunct to olanzapine treatment, and modest reductions in weight gain were seen in patients receiving 300 mg of nizatidine versus placebo; however, weight gain still occurred in these olanzapine-treated patients (Werneke et al. 2002). Metformin, an oral hypoglycemic agent utilized for treatment of type II diabetes that increases insulin sensitivity in insulin-resistant patients, may also be useful as a weight loss agent (Baptista et al. 2001; DeFronzo and Goodman 1995; Fontbonne et al. 1996; Morrison et al. 2002). Of course, caution must temper enthusiasm for the results from these small studies, and more prospective, better-powered intervention studies are desperately needed.

Conclusion

Obesity is a growing problem in the United States in the general population, and this epidemic also plagues our patients with schizophrenia. Antipsychotic medications, the illness itself, poverty, and lack of adequate medical care all contribute to overweight and obesity in this patient population. Mental health practitioners need to take the initiative to minimize this problem by initially choosing antipsychotic medications with more favorable weight gain profiles; rigorously monitoring weight and related parameters, such as blood glucose and lipids; and educating patients about diet and exercise to equip them with the skills to avoid obesity and its health consequences. Adjunctive pharmacological interventions for obesity in the chronically mentally ill population are as yet unproven, although they may prove to be helpful, but simple behavioral interventions should always be attempted to help patients lose weight and prevent the long-term morbidity and mortality associated with overweight and obesity.

References

Allison DB, Mentore JL, Heo M, et al: Antipsychotic-induced weight gain: a comprehensive research synthesis. Am J Psychiatry 156:1686–1696, 1999a

Allison D, Fontaine K, Moonseong H, et al: The distribution of body mass index among individuals with and without schizophrenia. J Clin Psychiatry 60:215–220, 1999b

Allison D, Mackell J: Healthcare resource use and body mass index among individuals with schizophrenia. Poster presented at the annual meeting of the New Clinical Drug Evaluation Unit, Boca Raton, FL, May 2000

Aronne LJ: Epidemiology, morbidity, and treatment of overweight and obesity. J Clin Psychiatry 62 (suppl 23):13–22, 2001

Aulakh CS, Hill JL, Yoney HT, et al: Evidence for involvement of 5-HT$_{1C}$ and 5-HT$_2$ receptors in the food intake suppressant effects of 1-(2,5-dimethoxy-4-iodophenyl)-2-aminopropane (DOI). Psychopharmacologia 109:444–448, 1992

Ball MP, Coons VB, Buchanan RW: A program for treating olanzapine-related weight gain. Psychiatr Serv 52:967–969, 2001

Baptista T, Hernandez L, Prieto LA, et al: Metformin in obesity associated with antipsychotic drug administration: a pilot study. J Clin Psychiatry 62:653–655, 2001

Basson BR, Kinon BJ, Taylor CC, et al: Factors influencing acute weight change in patients with schizophrenia treated with olanzapine, haloperidol or risperidone. J Clin Psychiatry 62:231–238, 2001

Bernstein JG: Psychotropic drug induced weight gain: mechanisms and management. Clin Neuropharmacol 11 (suppl 1):S194–S206, 1988

Berry SA, Mahmoud RA: Normalization of olanzapine associated abnormalities of insulin resistance and insulin release after switch to risperidone: the risperidone rescue study. Poster presented at the 40th annual meeting of the American College of Neuropsychopharmacology, Kona, HI, December 2001

Brecher M, Melvin K: Effect of long term quetiapine monotherapy on weight in schizophrenia. Poster presented at the annual meeting of the American Psychiatric Association, New Orleans, Louisiana, May 2001

Bromel T, Blum W, Ziegler A, et al: Serum leptin levels increase rapidly after initiation of clozapine treatment. Mol Psychiatry 3:76–80, 1998

Bustillo JR, Buchanan RW, Irish D, et al: Differential effect of clozapine on weight: a controlled study. Am J Psychiatry 153:817–819, 1996

Cerulli J, Lomaestro B, Malone M: Update on the pharmacotherapy of obesity. Ann Pharmacother 32:88–102, 1998

Colditz GA: Economic costs of obesity and inactivity. Med Sci Sports Exerc 31 (suppl 11):S663–S667, 1999

Correa N, Opler LA, Kay SR, et al: Amantadine in the treatment of neuroendocrine side effects of neuroleptics. J Clin Psychopharmacol 7:91–95, 1987

Davidson S, Judd F, Jolley D, et al: Cardiovascular risk factors for people with mental illness. Aust N Z J Psychiatry 35:196–202, 2001

DeFronzo RA, Goodman AM: Multicenter Metformin Study Group: efficacy of metformin in patients with non-insulin-dependent diabetes mellitus. N Engl J Med 333:541–549, 1995

Eder U, Mangweth B, Ebenbichler C, et al: Association of olanzapine-induced weight gain with an increase in body fat. Am J Psychiatry 158:1719–1722, 2001

Flegal KM, Troiano RP: Changes in the distribution of body mass index of adults and children in the US population. Int J Obes Relat Metab Disord 24:807–818, 2000

Fontaine KR, Heo M, Harrigan EP, et al: Estimating the consequences of antipsychotic induced weight gain on health and mortality rate. Psychiatry Res 101(3):277–288, 2001

Fontbonne A, Charles MA, Juhan-Vague I, et al: The effect of metformin on the metabolic abnormalities associated with upper-body fat distribution. Diabetes Care 19:920–926, 1996

Furst BA, Champion KM, Pierre JM, et al: Possible association of QTc interval prolongation with co-administration of quetiapine and lovastatin. Biol Psychiatry 51:264–265, 2002

Garattini S, Mennini T, Samain R: Reduction of food intake by manipulation of central serotonin: current experimental results. Br J Psychiatry 155 (suppl 8):41–51, 1989

Geodon. New York, Pfizer, 2001 [package insert]

Goodall E, Oxtoby C, Richards R, et al: A clinical trial of the efficacy and acceptability of D-fenfluramine in the treatment of neuroleptic-induced obesity. Br J Psychiatry 153:208–213, 1988

Green AI, Patel JK, Goisman RM, et al: Weight gain from novel antipsychotic drugs: need for action. Gen Hosp Psychiatry 22:224–235, 2000

Groop L, Orho-Melander M: The dysmetabolic syndrome. J Intern Med 250:105–120, 2001

Gupta S, Droney T, Al-Samarrai S, et al: Olanzapine: weight gain and therapeutic efficacy. J Clin Psychopharmacol 19:273–275, 1999

Henderson DC, Cagliero E, Gray C, et al: Clozapine, diabetes mellitus, weight gain, and lipid abnormalities: a five-year naturalistic study. Am J Psychiatry 157:975–981, 2000

Hilgar E, Quiner S, Ginzel I, et al: The effect of orlistat on plasma levels of psychotropic drugs in patients with long-term psychopharmacotherapy. J Clin Psychopharmacol 22:68–70, 2002

Jones AM, Rak IW, Raniwalla J, et al: Weight changes in patients treated with quetiapine. Poster presented at the annual meeting of the American Psychiatric Association, Chicago, IL, May 2000

Kingsbury SJ, Fayek M, Trufasiu D, et al: The apparent effects of ziprasidone on plasma lipids and glucose. J Clin Psychiatry 62:347–349, 2001

Kinon BJ, Basson BR, Gilmore JA, et al: Long-term olanzapine treatment: weight change and weight-related health factors in schizophrenia. J Clin Psychiatry 62:92–100, 2001

Knapp M: Schizophrenia costs and treatment cost-effectiveness. Acta Psychiatrica Scand Suppl 102:15–18, 2000

Knight A: Astemizole: a new, non-sedating antihistamine for hay fever. J Otolaryngol 14:85–88, 1985

Kolokowska T, Gadhvi H, Molyneux S: An open clinical trial of fenfluramine in chronic schizophrenia: a pilot study. Int Clin Psychopharmacol 2:83–88, 1987

Kraepelin E: Dementia Praecox and Paraphrenia. Edinburgh, E & S Livingstone, 1919

Kraus T, Haack M, Schuld A, et al: Body weight and leptin plasma levels during treatment with antipsychotic drugs. Am J Psychiatry 156:312–314, 1999

Leadbetter R, Shutty M, Pavalonis D, et al: Clozapine-induced weight gain: prevalence and clinical relevance. Am J Psychiatry 149:68–72, 1992

Luque C, Rey J: Sibutramine: a serotonin-norepinephrine reuptake-inhibitor for the treatment of obesity. Ann Pharmacother 33:968–978, 1999

Marder S, Davis JM, Chouinard G, et al: The effects of risperidone on the five dimensions of schizophrenia. J Clin Psychiatry 58:538–546, 1997

McElroy S, Suppes T, Keck P, et al: Open-label adjunctive topiramate in the treatment of bipolar disorders. Biol Psychiatry 47:1025–1033, 2000

McIntyre RS, Trakas K, Lin D, et al: Risk of adverse events associated with antipsychotic treatment: results from the Canadian National Outcomes Measurement Study in Schizophrenia (CNOMSS). Abstract presented at the 40th annual meeting of the American College of Neuropsychopharmacology, Kona, HI, December 2001

Meyer JM: Novel antipsychotics and severe hyperlipidemia. J Clin Psychopharmacol 21:369–374, 2001

Meyer JM: A retrospective comparison of lipid, glucose and weight changes at one year between olanzapine and risperidone treated inpatients. J Clin Psychiatry 63: 425–433, 2002

Mokdad AH, Ford ES, Bowman BA, et al: Diabetes trends in the U.S.: 1990–1998. Diabetes Care 23:1278–1283, 2000a

Mokdad AH, Serdula MK, Dietz WH, et al: The continuing epidemic of obesity in the United States. JAMA 284:1650–1651, 2000b

Morrison JA, Cottingham EM, Barton BA: Metformin for weight loss in pediatric patients taking psychotropic drugs. Am J Psychiatry 159:655–657, 2002

Must A, Spadano J, Coakley EH, et al: The disease burden associated with overweight and obesity. JAMA 282:1523–1529, 1999

Myers A, Rosen JC: Obesity stigmatizationa and coping: relation to mental health symptoms, body image, and self-esteem. Int J Obes Relat Metab Disord 23:221–230, 1999

National Heart, Lung and Blood Institute (NHLBI): Clinical guidelines on the identification, evaluation, and treatment of overweight and obesity in adults. Available at: http://www.nhlbi.nih.gov/guidelines/obesity/practgd_c.pdf. November 2000

Nemeroff CB: Dosing the antipsychotic medication olanzapine. J Clin Psychiatry 58 (suppl 10):45–49, 1997

Norton J, Potter D, Edward K: Sustained weight loss associated with topiramate. Epilepsia 38 (suppl 3):S60, 1997

Park YW, Allison DB, Heymsfield SB, et al: Larger amounts of visceral adipose tissue in Asian Americans. Obes Res 9:381–387, 2001

Pelleymounter M, Cullen M, Baker M, et al: Effects of the obese gene production body weight regulation in ob/ob mice. Science 269:240–243, 1995

Petrie J, Saha A, McEvoy J: Aripiprazole, a new atypical antipsychotic: phase II clinical trial result. Eur Neuropsychopharmacol 7 (suppl 2):S227, 1997

Pfizer: Briefing document for ziprasidone HCl presented at the FDA Psychopharmacological Drugs Advisory Committee, July 19, 2000

Reinstein M, Sirotovskaya L, Jonas L, et al: Effect of clozapine-quetiapine combination therapy on weight and glycaemic control. Clin Drug Invest 18:99–104, 1999

Risperdal. Titusville, NJ, Janssen Pharmaceutica, 1999 [package insert]

Rockwell WJ, Ellinwood EH, Trader DW: Psychotropic drugs promoting weight gain: health risks and treatment implications. South Med J 76:1407–1412, 1983

Rosenfeld W, Schaefer P, Pace K: Weight loss patterns with topiramate therapy. Epilepsia 38 (suppl 3):S58, 1997

Rotatori AF, Fox R, Wicks A: Weight loss with psychiatric residents in a behavioral self-control program. Psychol Rep 46:483–486, 1980

Sacchetti E, Guarner L, Bravi D: H_2 antagonist nizatidine may control olanzapine-associated weight gain in schizophrenic patients. Biol Psychiatry 48:167–168, 2000

Samanin R, Garattini S: The pharmacology of serotonergic drugs affecting appetite, in Nutrition and the Brain, Vol 8. Edited by Wurtman RJ, Wurtman JJ. New York, Raven, 1990, pp 163–192

Schlosser E: Fast Food Nation: The Dark Side of the All-American Meal. Boston, Houghton Mifflin, 2001

Schotte A, Janssen PF, Megens AA, et al: Occupancy of central neurotransmitter receptors by risperidone, clozapine, and haloperidol measured ex vivo by quantitative autoradiography. Brain Res 631:191–202, 1993

Seroquel. Wilmington, DE, AstraZeneca, 2000 [package insert]

Silverstone T, Smith G, Goodall E: Prevalence of obesity in patients receiving depot antipsychotics. Br J Psychiatry 153:214–217, 1988

Taylor DM, McAskill R: Atypical antipsychotics and weight gain: a systematic review. Acta Psychiatr Scand 101:416–432, 2000

Tecott L, Sun L, Arkana S: Eating disorder and epilepsy in mice lacking $5\text{-}HT_{2C}$ serotonin receptors. Nature 374:542–546, 1995

Theisen FM, Linden A, Geller F, et al: Prevalence of obesity in adolescent and young adult patients with and without schizophrenia and in relationship to antipsychotic medication. J Psychiatr Res 35:339–345, 2001

Umbricht DS, Pollack S, Kane JM: Clozapine and weight gain. J Clin Psychiatry 55 (suppl B):157–160, 1994

Weiden PJ, Allison DB, Mackell JA, et al: Obesity as a risk factor for antipsychotic noncompliance. Poster presented at the annual meeting of the American Psychiatric Association, Chicago, IL, May 2000

Werneke U, Taylor D, Sanders TA: Options for pharmacological treatment of obesity in patients treated with atypical antipsychotics. Int Clin Psychopharmacol 17:145–160, 2002

Wirshing D, Wirshing W, Kysar L, et al: Novel antipsychotics:comparison of weight gain liabilities. J Clin Psychiatry 60:358–363, 1999

Wirshing DA, Pierre JM, Eyeler J, et al: Risperidone associated new-onset diabetes. Biol Psychiatry 50:1489–1489, 2001a

Wirshing D, Boyd J, Meng L, et al: Antipsychotic medication: impact on coronary artery disease risk factors. Biol Psychiatry 49:175S, 2001b

Wolf A, Colditz G: Current estimates of the economic cost of obesity in the United States. Obes Res 6:97–106, 1998

Yanovski J, Yanovski S: Recent advances in basic obesity research. JAMA 282:1504–1506, 1999

Yanovski S, Yanovski J: Obesity. N Engl J Med 346:591–602, 2002

Zyprexa. Indianapolis, IN, Eli Lilly, 2000 [package insert]

Chapter 4

Cardiovascular Illness and Hyperlipidemia in Patients With Schizophrenia

Jonathan M. Meyer, M.D.

Introduction

In Westernized societies, cardiovascular disease is a significant cause of medical morbidity and mortality, a trend that emerged in the first half of the twentieth century as the percentage of deaths from cardiovascular disease increased in the United States to 50% of the population from only 15% in 1900 (Pearson and Boden 2000). Although mortality from coronary heart disease (CHD) has declined significantly since that time due to the advent of coronary care units, the development of reperfusion and stent technologies, widespread availability of defibrillators, and the use of aspirin, statin therapy, and beta-blockers, the overall incidence of cardiovascular disease in the United States has steadily increased, with no reductions in the number of individuals with established coronary heart disease noted over the past decade. In part this is due to the dramatic increase in the prevalence of overweight and obesity, with a concomitant rise in the number of individuals with diabetes (Flegal and Troiano 2000).

Approximately 70% of coronary disease mortality can be accounted for by the so-called traditional risk factors of hypertension, smoking, diabetes mellitus, and hyperlipidemia, conditions with particular relevance for patients with schizophrenia due to their higher-than-normal prevalence in this population. Therefore, for patients with schizophrenia, a common medical sequela is the development of cardiovascular disease in a proportion greater than that found among the general population. A meta-analysis of mortality studies published from 1952 through 1996 found standardized mortality ratios (SMRs) for cardiovascular disorders of 1.12 for males and 1.09 for females with schizophrenia, both of which were statistically significant. More recent data published by Brown et al. (2000) calculated the SMR for cardiovascular disorders on a cohort of 370 patients with schizophrenia followed for 13 years, and found that these patients were nearly 2.5 times more likely to die of a circulatory cause than those in the general population (males 2.62, females 2.30). A similar relative risk for cardiovascular mortality of 2.2 was noted among a sample of 3,022 Canadian patients with schizophrenia followed for 39 months compared with 12,088 age- and gender-matched control subjects (Curkendall et al. 2001). These higher figures are corroborated by the data generated from Osby et al. (2000) in their comprehensive study of 7,784 persons admitted with schizophrenia in Stockholm from 1973 to 1995. The cardiovascular SMRs in that population were 2.3 and 2.1 for males and females, respectively. More important, the largest single cause of death in both males and females was cardiovascular disease followed by suicide, with cardiovascular disease also the main cause of excess deaths in females.

The excess mortality from cardiovascular causes in patients with schizophrenia is not entirely unexpected, given the prevalence of underlying risk factors such as sedentary lifestyle, obesity, smoking, and glucose intolerance (the latter three of which are discussed at length in this volume in Chapters 2, 5, and 6, respectively). The development of cardiovascular disease has a significant negative impact on quality of life, particularly among the chronically mentally ill, who often have limited access to general medical services. In open systems, such as the Veterans Affairs (VA) hospitals and clinics, where barriers to access are relatively few, the use of cholesterol-lowering agents in those with schizophrenia who see a primary care provider is comparable to their use in those without major mental illness; yet a substantial fraction of patients receiving psychiatric care at VA clinics do not receive routine primary care (Dollarhide, Matthews, Cadenhead, unpublished data; Druss et al. 2001). Once access is gained, the utilization of interventions such as cardiac catheterization following myocardial infarction (MI) is 41% lower in patients with schizophrenia than among those without mental disorder (Druss et al. 2000).

The chronically mentally ill thus represent a vulnerable population for the development of cardiovascular disease mainly due to lifestyle-related risk factors, but emerging data now also implicate the use of certain classes of antipsychotics as significant contributors to cardiovascular risk through their metabolic side effects—namely, weight gain, impairment of glucose tolerance, and hyperlipidemia (McIntyre et al. 2001). During therapy of patients with schizophrenia, mental health practitioners are not primarily focused on the substantial cardiovascular risk imposed by hyperlipidemia, and they may therefore be disinclined to perform lipid monitoring in patients prescribed antipsychotics associated with hyperlipidemia or to refer patients for lipid-lowering therapy. Given the immediately observable psychiatric benefits of antipsychotic therapy, the health risks imposed by hyperlipidemia become a secondary issue. Mental health providers should not feel unduly chastened in this regard, because data indicate that even among patients with documented CHD seen by primary care providers, only 14% receive lipid-lowering therapy when indicated, and only 18% ever achieve their target serum lipid goals (Hoerger et al. 1998; Pearson 2000).

The purpose of this chapter is to review the data on cardiovascular risk as they apply to patients with schizophrenia, particularly the role of hyperlipidemia; to discuss the literature relating antipsychotic therapy to changes in serum lipids; and to equip mental health providers with a useful set of tools for screening chronically mentally ill clients for cardiovascular risk factors, including appropriate lipid-monitoring strategies during antipsychotic therapy, and a simple method for quantifying cardiovascular risk.

Risk Factors for Cardiovascular Illness and Their Prevalence in Patients With Schizophrenia

As with many chronic disorders, prevention is the key, and patients with schizophrenia possess numerous modifiable cardiovascular risk factors that may be the focus of intervention. As Osby et al. (2000) concluded, "The number of excess deaths, rather than increased SMRs, may be the target for preventive programs since the aim of prevention should be to reduce this excess mortality" (p. 25). The literature on cardiovascular risk factors is rapidly evolving, but a core group of modifiable risk factors have emerged as targets for treatment (Table 4–1). Individuals at risk present with a constellation of modifiable and nonmodifiable risk factors, with the latter including age, gender, family history, personal history, and genetic predisposition toward high CHD risk by various mechanisms inducing

Table 4–1.   Modifiable risk factors for cardiovascular disease and their prevalence in patients with schizophrenia

Risk factor	Prevalence in schizophrenia (%)
Elevated total cholesterol	≥18
Hypertension	13.7–19.7
Smoking	70
Overweight or obesity	42–55
Sedentary lifestyle	72

obesity, dyslipidemias, and diabetes mellitus. Although the prevalence of most modifiable CHD risk factors in schizophrenia is higher than in the general population, there is no evidence that patients with schizophrenia are genetically predisposed to cardiovascular disease in a manner not explicable by traditional risk factor analysis. There are two lines of evidence to support this conclusion. Postmortem evaluation of schizophrenic patients earlier this century demonstrated findings of hypoplasia of the heart and great vessels, but recent necropsy studies, such as that by Coffman et al., that exclude patients with known cardiovascular diseases have not found statistically significant differences in measures of left atrial, aortic root, or end-diastolic left ventricular diameter (Coffman et al. 1985). Moreover, reviews of sudden-death cases involving patients with schizophrenia reveal that typical natural causes such as atherosclerotic cardiovascular disease constitute the majority of etiologies once suicide and accidents are excluded (Chute et al. 1999; Ruschena et al. 1998).

The current understanding of cardiovascular risk factors comes from large, longitudinal epidemiological studies such as the Framingham Heart Study (Wilson et al. 1988) and the Multiple Risk Factor Intervention Trial (MRFIT; Stamler et al. 1986). These studies have helped elucidate the contributions of age, family history of CHD, gender, smoking, overweight and obesity, diabetes, hypertension, diet, lifestyle, and serum cholesterol to overall cardiovascular risk. In particular, MRFIT, a longitudinal 6-year study of 356,222 individuals, demonstrated the linear relationship between serum cholesterol and CHD deaths. Biological effects independent of lifestyle variables (e.g., smoking, activity, diet) thus contribute on average approximately 40%–60% to overall CHD risk (Engstrom et al. 2000). Those in the highest risk group are persons with established CHD or equivalent disorders, defined as those pathologies that, along with established CHD, exhibit a >20% 10-year risk for major coronary events such as fatal or nonfatal MI, unstable angina, or sudden death. These CHD equivalent disorders include diabetes mellitus and other clinical forms of atherosclerotic disease (peripheral arterial disease, abdominal aortic aneurysm, and symptomatic carotid artery disease). The National Cholesterol Education Program (NCEP) published its third series of revised guidelines for management of cholesterol and cardiovascular risk in 2001, and included diabetes as a CHD equivalent for the following reason: "Diabetes counts as a CHD risk equivalent because it confers a high risk of new CHD within 10 years, in part because of its frequent association with multiple risk factors. Furthermore, because persons with diabetes who experience MI have unusually high death rates either immediately or in the long term, a more intensive prevention strategy is warranted" (Expert Panel on Detection, Evaluation, and Treatment of High Blood Cholesterol in Adults 2001, p. 2487).

For those without established CHD or CHD equivalent disorders, 10-year cardiovascular risk estimates can be performed quite simply with a risk chart such as that created by the NCEP on the basis of data from the Framingham study and trials of lipid-lowering agents (Table 4–2). These charts are gender specific and use data on age, smoking status, systolic blood pressure, and both total serum cholesterol and high-density lipoprotein (HDL) cholesterol to generate the risk estimate for a major coronary event over the next decade. Points are assigned to each risk factor, and total points are converted to risk estimates expressed in percentages.

Obesity

Overweight and obesity, although recognized independent risk factors for CHD, are typically not included in coronary risk charts (Jones et al. 2001). One rationale for this is that obesity has significant comorbidity with hypertension, hyperlipidemia, and glucose intolerance, and in that sense it becomes a surrogate marker for these disorders with well-defined risk parameters. Nevertheless, the plateau in CHD prevalence in the United States is attributed in large measure to the epidemic of obesity, with nearly 27% of the population registering a body mass index greater than 30 kg/m^2, the established cutoff for defining obesity (Flegal and Troiano 2000). This figure is 80% greater than that noted two decades prior. Longitudinal data, such as the 18-year Nijmegen Cohort Study, which examined changes in serum total cholesterol levels in a cohort of men and women, clearly demonstrate that weight gain correlates over time with increased cholesterol, and weight gain itself exerts a significantly greater influence on the rise in serum cholesterol than does initial body weight (Bakx et al. 2000). The distribution of weight gain is also increasingly recognized as an important independent risk factor for significant metabolic and atherosclerotic disease because of

Table 4–2. Ten-year Framingham cardiovascular risk estimation charts

Males

Age	Points
20–34	–9
35–39	–4
40–44	0
45–49	3
50–54	6
55–59	8
60–64	10
65–69	11
70–74	12
75–79	13

Total cholesterol (mg/dL)	Points				
	Age 20–39	Age 40–49	Age 50–59	Age 60–69	Age 70–79
<160	0	0	0	0	0
160–199	4	3	2	1	1
200–239	7	5	3	1	0
240–279	9	6	4	2	1
≥280	11	8	5	3	1

	Points				
	Age 20–39	Age 40–49	Age 50–59	Age 60–69	Age 70–79
Nonsmoker	0	0	0	0	0
Smoker	8	5	3	1	1

HDL (mg/dL)	Points
≥60	–1
50–59	0
40–49	1
<40	2

Systolic BP (mm Hg)	If untreated	If treated
<120	0	0
120–129	0	1
130–139	1	2
140–159	1	2
≥160	2	3

Point total	10-year cardiovascular risk (%)
<0	<1
0–4	1
5	2
6	2
7	3
8	4
9	5
10	6
11	8
12	10
13	12
14	16
15	20
16	25
≥17	≥30

Source. Expert Panel. JAMA 285:2486–2489, 2001.

Table 4–2. Ten-year Framingham cardiovascular risk estimation charts *(continued)*

Females

Age	Points
20–34	−7
35–39	−3
40–44	0
45–49	3
50–54	6
55–59	8
60–64	10
65–69	12
70–74	14
75–79	16

Total cholesterol (mg/dL)	Points				
	Age 20–39	Age 40–49	Age 50–59	Age 60–69	Age 70–79
<160	0	0	0	0	0
160–199	4	3	2	1	1
200–239	8	6	4	2	1
240–279	11	8	5	3	2
≥280	13	10	7	4	2

	Points				
	Age 20–39	Age 40–49	Age 50–59	Age 60–69	Age 70–79
Nonsmoker	0	0	0	0	0
Smoker	9	7	4	2	1

HDL (mg/dL)	Points
≥60	−1
50–59	0
40–49	1
<40	2

Systolic BP (mm Hg)	If untreated	If treated
<120	0	0
120–129	1	3
130–139	2	4
140–159	3	5
≥160	4	6

Point total	10-year cardiovascular risk (%)
<9	<1
9–12	1
13	2
14	2
15	3
16	4
17	5
18	6
19	8
20	11
21	14
22	17
23	22
24	27
≥25	≥30

Note. HDL=high-density lipoprotein; BP=blood pressure.

the association between truncal obesity and the metabolic syndrome, or syndrome X, which comprises a cluster of abnormalities including abdominal obesity, dyslipidemia with elevated triglycerides and low HDL cholesterol, hypertension, hypercoagulability, and evidence of insulin resistance (with or without overt glucose intolerance) (Bard et al. 2001; Grundy 1999). An estimated 22% of adults in the United States meet criteria for the metabolic syndrome, making this an intense focus of research among epidemiologists and clinicians (Ford et al. 2002).

Although obesity is not included in coronary risk charts for the aforementioned reasons, the association between obesity and cardiovascular disease is indeed strong, with compelling data demonstrating that even modest amounts of weight loss (e.g., 8.5% of body mass) may achieve significant benefits in cardiovascular risk, in part due to favorable effects on serum lipids and glucose homeostasis (Melanson et al. 2001; Rossner et al. 2000). A return to ideal body weight may reduce overall cardiovascular risk as much as 35%–55% (Wood and Joint European Societies Task 2001). Of particular relevance is the fact that recent estimates of obesity prevalence among patients with schizophrenia are 1.5 to 2 times that for the general population (Allison and Casey 2001; Allison et al. 1999a). The trend toward overweight and obesity was present among patients with schizophrenia, particularly females, prior to the advent of atypical antipsychotics, but the concern has increased dramatically over the past 5 years due to evidence of profound weight gain with certain atypical antipsychotics, particularly olanzapine and clozapine, to an extent much greater than that achieved even with low-potency typical agents such as chlorpromazine (Allison et al. 1999b; Blackburn 2000; Meyer 2001a). Moreover, the weight gain from atypical antipsychotics is primarily in the form of greater adiposity, not increases in lean muscle mass (Eder et al. 2001).

Smoking

Smoking cessation continues to be a primary focus of lifestyle modification aimed at reduction of cardiovascular risk because of the powerful association between smoking and CHD. A meta-analysis of prospective epidemiological studies spanning four decades of research established the relative risk for cardiovascular disease among smokers of 20 cigarettes per day at 1.78 (Law et al. 1997). The range of relative risk varies with age and is 4.46 at age 45, 3.07 at age 55, 1.78 at age 65, and 1.34 at age 75. Even among those who smoke only 1 cigarette per day, the relative risk of CHD compared with those who never smoke ranges from 1.93 at age 45 to 1.39 at age 65. Utilizing an epidemiological risk estimation method known as rate advancement period, one can calculate that, on average, smokers are expected to advance their risk of MI by approximately 11 years compared with never or former smokers (Liese et al. 2000). Discontinuing smoking may thereby reduce the risk of CHD by as much as 50%, with the overall risk returning to that of the general population after 20 years of abstinence (Eliasson et al. 2001; Villablanca et al. 2000). The relationship between smoking and CHD derives from numerous chemicals in cigarette smoke that act via multiple mechanisms to cause atherosclerosis, vascular injury, and increased coagulability (Villablanca et al. 2000). Limited exposure to such chemicals in the form of passive environmental smoke can increase the risk of cardiovascular disease as much as 30% (Smith et al. 2000).

Patients with schizophrenia have a prevalence rate of smoking nearly twice that of the general population, with estimates of 58%–88% in outpatient groups, and 79% or more in chronic inpatient settings (de Leon et al. 1995; Kelly and McCreadie 1999; Hughes et al. 1986). The connections between nicotine, smoking behavior, and schizophrenia are covered extensively in Chapter 5 of this volume, but it is worthwhile to note that those with schizophrenia not only have a higher prevalence of smoking, but also smoke more cigarettes on average, and more deeply, thereby increasing their exposure to mutagens and other noxious elements in cigarette smoke (Olincy et al. 1997). As a contributing risk factor for CHD, smoking remains the single most important lifestyle variable, and the greatest contributor to excess mortality from cardiovascular causes.

Hypertension

Hypertension does not appear to be more prevalent in patients with schizophrenia, although data are conflicting in this regard. One recent cross-sectional study of cardiovascular risk factors among 234 outpatients with schizophrenia in Melbourne, Australia, found no significant difference in the prevalence of hypertension compared with the general population (Davidson et al. 2001). Curkendall and colleagues' study of 3,022 Canadian patients with schizophrenia (mean age 49.6 years) found a 13.7% prevalence of hypertension, compared with a 16.7% prevalence noted in age- and gender-matched control subjects (Curkendall et al. 2001). The latter is comparable to the 15% prevalence obtained by a chart review of 179 state hospital patients in upstate New York (Bellnier et al. 2001). However, Cohn's naturalistic study of 133 long-term Canadian inpatients found a prevalence of hypertension in males and females of 28% and 24%, respectively, which was significantly greater than the values of 16% and 13% for male and female age- and gender-matched control subjects (Cohn and Remington 2001).

Similarly, the Patient Outcomes Research Team (PORT) study of 719 persons with schizophrenia found that 34.1% reported having been given a diagnosis of hypertension at some time by a physician, although only 19.7% stated that they currently had hypertension at the time of the survey (Dixon et al. 1999). Although patients with schizophrenia are prone to undertreatment of medical illnesses, 80.6% of those with active hypertension at time of survey were receiving antihypertensive therapy.

As with the other established risk factors, the association between hypertension and CHD has been elucidated through results of large, prospective clinical trials. The Nijmegen Cohort Study, a prospective cohort study of 7,092 Caucasian men and women with an 18-year follow-up, revealed that both systolic and diastolic blood pressure were independently associated with the likelihood of developing CHD. The significant risk ratios for systolic hypertension were 1.6 for men and 2.1 for women, and for diastolic hypertension 1.4 for men and 2.0 for women (Bakx et al. 2001). Data from a 32-year prospective follow-up study of 3,267 initially healthy male business executives showed that total mortality curves of the whole cohort increased significantly beyond 140 mm Hg systolic or 85 mm Hg diastolic (Strandberg et al. 2001). The impact of hypertension on CHD mortality is such that in patients with untreated hypertension and hyperlipidemia, starting antihypertensive therapy in those ages 35–74 results in a greater net reduction in deaths from coronary artery disease than lipid-lowering treatment alone (Perreault et al. 1999).

Diabetes

The importance of diabetes mellitus (DM) as an independent risk factor for CHD is such that the most recent version of the NCEP guidelines has raised DM to the category of a disease equivalent in long-term risk for major coronary events to having established CHD (Expert Panel on Detection, Evaluation, and Treatment of High Blood Cholesterol in Adults 2001). Of greater concern is the fact that modest levels of glucose intolerance that do not fall into the diabetic range (fasting glucose 126 mg/dL or greater) can substantially increase the risk for CHD and coronary events. Data from a metaregression analysis of 20 published studies comprising 95,783 individuals followed for 12.4 years revealed that even modest glucose intolerance among nondiabetics (mean fasting glucose 110 mg/dL) increases risk of cardiovascular events 33% compared with those with fasting glucose of 75 mg/dL (Coutinho et al. 1999). A case-control study among nondiabetic Southeast Asians found that, compared to patients whose fasting glucose was under 81 mg/dL, patients with fasting glucose between 95 and 114 mg/dL had over three times the relative risk for MI (Gerstein et al. 1999). Studies employing other peripheral markers of glucose intolerance in nondiabetic patients reveal similar trends (Gerstein et al. 2001).

These data are profoundly concerning for two reasons: 1) The prevalence of DM among patients with schizophrenia is approximately twice that in the general population (Curkendall et al. 2001; Dixon et al. 2000); and 2) there is an association between the use of certain atypical antipsychotics, especially the dibenzodiazepine compounds clozapine and olanzapine, and the development of glucose intolerance or new-onset DM during therapy, at times not associated with significant increases in weight (Haupt et al. 2001; Henderson et al. 2000; McIntyre et al. 2001). Thus, the finding that patients on olanzapine may experience a 10 mg/dL increase in fasting glucose after one year of treatment implies a significant rise in cardiovascular risk (Meyer 2002). The greatest risk is achieved once the patient meets the criteria for diabetes, with long-term data indicating an incidence of new-onset DM in patients exposed to olanzapine or clozapine of 7% per year (Casey 2000; Henderson et al. 2000).

Lifestyle Factors

Patients with schizophrenia are predisposed to lower levels of physical activity due the combined effects of sedating psychotropic medications and the core negative symptoms of the illness itself. Among the 234 outpatients with schizophrenia in Melbourne surveyed by Davidson and colleagues, participants were half as likely to undertake light exercise (odds ratio [OR] 0.54, 95% confidence interval [CI] 0.39–0.77), and one-fourth as likely to engage in vigorous exercise (OR=0.26, 95% CI=0.17–0.39) (Davidson et al. 2001). Seventy-two percent of a sample of 529 patients with schizophrenia or schizoaffective disorder screened for a medication trial reported having a sedentary lifestyle (Ascher-Svanum et al. 2001). Not surprisingly, there is an inverse linear dose relationship between moderate exercise and both all-cause mortality and CHD risk documented in numerous studies (Kohl 2001). The Iowa Study of 40,417 women ages 55–69 followed for 7 years showed that engaging in long walks, gardening, or light sport activities only four times per week decreased cardiovascular mortality by 47%. The Nurses Health Study of 72,488 women ages 40–65 followed for 8 years showed a 33% reduction in cardiovascular deaths for those in the most active group (Wannamethee and Shaper 2001). Thus, one need only engage in 2–3 hours per week of moderate exercise to achieve significant reduction in CHD-related mortality. What is not clear is whether vigorous activity confers additional benefit beyond that achieved through moderate exercise (Lee and Skerrett 2001).

Another important lifestyle factor that contributes to CHD risk is diet, particularly high intake of saturated fat (Hooper et al. 2001) and low intake of fiber or unsaturated fats (Kromhout 2001; Pereira and Pins 2000). Data from the Framingham Heart Study accrued over 50 years have clarified the importance of a balanced diet as a preventive measure for CHD (Millen and Quatromoni 2001). A comprehensive dietary intervention study performed in Finland aimed at cardiovascular disease risk reduction by altering the type of fats consumed, lowering sodium intake, and increasing vegetable and fruit consumption achieved dramatic reductions in cardiovascular mortality during the period 1972–1997, along with significant improvements in blood pressure and serum cholesterol levels (Pietinen et al. 2001). Although antioxidants are quite popular as health care supplements, there is no convincing evidence that either vitamin E, carotenoids, or vitamin C protect against CHD. Multiple studies seem to indicate that changing the total dietary profile is the intervention that will most consistently improve multiple cardiovascular risk factors, including hyperlipidemia, hypertension, glucose intolerance, and overweight or obesity (McCarron and Reusser 2000).

There is compelling evidence that patients with schizophrenia partake of a diet higher in fat and lower in fiber than that of the general population. At the end of a 15-year longitudinal study of patients with schizophrenia residing near Oxford, England, 132 out of 140 surviving participants (initial n of 175) were queried about lifestyle habits including intake of dietary fiber and fat (Brown et al. 1999). Significant differences were found in the amount of dietary fiber consumed ($P<0.001$) and total fat ($P=0.03$), but not intake of unsaturated fat ($P=0.19$). This study also found a lower prevalence of exercise than in the general age-matched population.

The use of alcohol is another lifestyle factor contributing to cardiovascular risk (Marques-Vidal et al. 2001). (The use of alcohol in patients with schizophrenia is covered extensively in Chapter 9 of this volume.) Nonetheless, it is worthwhile to note here that whereas Bellnier found that 49% of his state hospital patients reported a history of alcohol abuse, Davidson's data indicated that patients with schizophrenia may be both more likely to abstain from alcohol than the general population (OR=2.0, 95% CI=1.5–2.5) and to drink excessively compared with the general population (OR=4.0, 95% CI=2.7–6.0) (Davidson et al. 2001).

Hyperlipidemia

A complete review of lipid physiology is beyond the scope of this chapter; however, it is worth noting that the major classes of lipoproteins are divided on the basis of their weight under centrifugation (Kwiterovich 2000). The lightest are chylomicrons, derived from dietary triglycerides, and very-low-density lipoproteins (VLDL), which are endogenously produced triglyceride-rich particles; the next heavier particles are low-density lipoproteins (LDL) and high-density lipoproteins (HDL). Total cholesterol (TC) as obtained on a lipid panel reflects the combination of serum concentrations of VLDL (calculated as serum triglyceride levels divided by 5), LDL, and HDL. Normal serum TC concentration is defined as a fasting level under 200 mg/dL, normal HDL as ≥40 mg/dL, and the ideal serum LDL concentration determined by CV risk factors as noted later. The rate-limiting step in cholesterol synthesis is a reaction catalyzed by the enzyme 3-hydroxy-3-methylglutaryl coenzyme A (HMG CoA) reductase, the target for a class of lipid-lowering agents called statins. The MRFIT study clearly established the linear association between CHD and serum cholesterol, but further research clarified that risk is more properly associated with abnormalities involving the LDL and HDL cholesterol fractions, and separately by serum triglycerides (Stamler et al. 1986).

A series of landmark studies published in the mid-1990s demonstrated the significant association between reduction in LDL levels and reduced CV events and mortality. The Scandinavian Simvastatin Survival Study was a randomized, double-blind, placebo-controlled trial of cholesterol lowering in 4,444 patients with CHD already on a lipid-lowering diet, followed for a median of 5.4 years (Scandinavian Simvastatin Survival Study 1994). This secondary prevention study found that statin therapy reduced TC by 28% and LDL by 38%, with a 42% reduction in coronary deaths and 30% decrease in all-cause mortality compared with the placebo cohort. Another randomized, double-blind, placebo-controlled secondary prevention trial of pravastatin in 9,014 patients (ages 31–75) with ischemic heart disease followed for 6.1 years on average showed a 24% reduction in nonfatal MI or death due to CHD (LIPID Study Group 1998). A similar 24% reduction in nonfatal MI or death due to CHD was seen in a randomized, double-blind, placebo-controlled secondary prevention trial of pravaststin (n = 4,159) with patients after MI who had normal cholesterol levels (Sacks et al. 1996). Moreover, two primary prevention studies of patients without CHD but with either hypercholesterolemia or low HDL levels and average TC identified profound benefits from statin therapy. The West of Scotland Coronary Prevention Study (WOSCOPS) was a randomized, double-blind, placebo-controlled trial of pravastatin in 6,595 men, 45 to 64 years of age, with mean TC of 272 mg/dL and no history of MI, followed for a mean of 4.9 years (Shepherd et al. 1995). A 32% reduction in the development of CHD and a 22% reduction in total mortality was found in this tria. The Air Force/ Texas Coronary Atherosclerosis Prevention Study (AFCAPS/TEXCAPS) was a primary prevention trial of lovastatin versus placebo in men and women with no clinical evidence of cardiovascular disease, average total cholesterol and LDL levels, and low HDL (Downs et al. 1998). Over the 5.2 years of this study there was a 37% reduction in risk of major coronary events compared with the placebo group.

The revised 2001 NCEP guidelines used the results of these and other studies to establish LDL goals based on the number of underlying major cardiovascular risk factors: smoking, hypertension (blood pressure ≥140/90 mm Hg or on antihypertensive medication), low HDL cholesterol (<40 mg/dL), family history of premature CHD (CHD in male first-degree relative <55 years or female first-degree relative <65 years), and age (men ≥45 years, women ≥55 years). For those with zero or one risk factor the fasting LDL goal is <160 mg/dL, two or more risk factors <130 mg/dL, and those with CHD or CHD equivalent disorders (e.g., DM) <100 mg/dL. As of 2002, LDL continues to be the main focus of lipid-lowering therapy due to the powerful evidence from multiple large studies, although there are significant data from the Framingham Heart Study showing a 2%–4% increase in risk of CHD-related death for each 1 mg/dL decrease in HDL, with over 30% of deaths occurring in those with normal TC values (Wilson et al. 1988). As data accrue from other placebo-controlled studies focusing on increasing HDL, such as AFCAPS/ TEXCAPS, future guidelines may consider treatment of both LDL and HDL abnormalities as primary goals. Serum triglyceride concentrations are considered a secondary focus of lipid-lowering treatment, with clear evidence from several studies linking elevated triglyceride concentrations (i.e., ≥200 mg/dL) to increased CHD risk (Cullen 2000; Jeppesen et al. 1998; Rubins 2000). The importance of hypertriglyceridemia as a cardiovascular risk factor for this discussion relates to data reviewed in the next section that demonstrate an association between elevated triglyceride concentration and atypical antipsychotic therapy, especially with the dibenzodiazepine-derived compounds clozapine, olanzapine, and quetiapine (a dibenzothiazepine).

The prevalence of hyperlipidemia in schizophrenic patients is not well known because many patients do not obtain screening for lipid disorders. Davidson found that 64% of men in his survey study were unaware of their serum cholesterol compared with 53% in the general population, although 48% of female patients with schizophrenia had received cholesterol measurement compared with 38% in the general population (Davidson et al. 2001). Bellnier noted only 18% of a state hospital cohort received a diagnosis of hyperlipidemia, yet Meyer's study of chronic state hospital patients found that 46% on risperidone ($n=39$) and 60% on olanzapine ($n=37$) therapy had elevated fasting TC after 1 year of treatment, with 44% and 51% of risperidone- and olanzapine-treated patients, respectively, manifesting elevated triglyceride concentrations (Bellnier et al.

2001; Meyer 2002). Meyer's prevalence data are similar to those found by Cohn, who noted that 35% of chronic inpatients with schizophrenia had low fasting HDL and 36% had elevated triglyceride concentrations, both of which were significantly different from the control population ($P<0.01$), although there were no significant differences in the prevalence of hypercholesterolemia (43% vs. 40% in control subjects) or elevated LDL (8.6% vs. 14% in control subjects) (Cohn and Remington 2001).

Effects of Antipsychotics on Serum Lipids

Serum lipid levels may be influenced by multiple factors, including genetics, diet, weight gain, systemic illness (e.g., DM), and exogenous agents including alcohol and medications. An extensive list of medications from disparate drug classes exists, with each agent associated with a specific pattern of hyperlipidemia (Mantel-Teeuwisse et al. 2001). In many instances, the underlying mechanism effecting this change in lipid metabolism is unknown, as is the case with the hyperlipidemia associated with antipsychotic therapy. Typically, changes in serum lipids were not a focus of clinical antipsychotic trials, but the increased interest in health outcomes for patients with schizophrenia has resulted in a number of abstracts, published case series, and small studies examining the effects of antipsychotics, particularly atypical agents, on lipid profiles.

Typical Antipsychotics

Although typical antipsychotics exert their effects through a common mechanism of potent antagonism of dopamine D_2 receptors, treatment with the phenothiazine class of antipsychotics such as chlorpromazine or fluphenazine was associated with significant effects on serum lipids in a manner not seen during therapy with butyrophenones such as haloperidol. In the decade following the widespread availability of chlorpromazine, literature emerged documenting effects on lipids (Clark et al. 1967; Mefferd et al. 1958), but the specific effects on cholesterol fractions were not elucidated until the mid-1980s with Sasaki's data on phenothiazine-treated chronic inpatients (Sasaki et al. 1984). This study found that HDL levels were significantly lower ($P<0.001$) compared with normal control subjects, while the serum triglyceride level was significantly higher ($P<0.05$) in these phenothiazine-treated patients. In one subgroup of eight new patients with schizophrenia, serum HDL level decreased by 24%

within 1 week following phenothiazine administration. A follow-up study comparing patients on phenothiazines with those receiving butyrophenones noted no significant differences in levels of total cholesterol, LDL, or HDL, yet the serum triglyceride level in patients receiving phenothiazines was 60% higher than in patients receiving butyrophenones (Sasaki et al. 1985). This finding of lipid neutrality for butyrophenones confirmed earlier data from the 1960s demonstrating either no effect of this antipsychotic class on TC and triglyceride concentration, or occasionally a small decrease in TC (Braun and Paulonis 1967; Simpson and Cooper 1966; Simpson et al. 1967).

Atypical Antipsychotics

While atypical antipsychotics share common pharmacodynamic properties, namely, potent antagonism of serotonin $5-HT_2$ receptors and weaker dopamine D_2 antagonism than typical agents, there are differential effects on serum lipids depending on the underlying chemical structure. What has emerged from data released over the past decade is the association between use of a dibenzodiazepine-derived atypical antipsychotic (i.e., clozapine, olanzapine, quetiapine) and profound effects on serum triglyceride levels, far greater than those seen during treatment with phenothiazine derivatives. This association between dibenzodiazepine structure and hypertriglyceridemia had emerged as early as 1986 with clinical studies of fluperlapine, a compound modeled on clozapine, in which severe elevations of serum triglyceride were noted, with one patient reaching a triglyceride concentration level of 900 mg/dL after 1 week of therapy (Fleischhacker et al. 1986; Muller-Oerlinghausen 1984). The first significant data on clozapine revealed that patients treated for 1 year had mean fasting serum triglyceride concentration of 264.0 mg/dL, compared with 149.8 mg/dL for those on typical agents, with three individuals in the clozapine cohort registering serum triglyceride levels greater than 500 mg/dL; however, there was no significant effect on TC (clozapine 217.0 mg/dL vs. typical 215.0 mg/dL) (Ghaeli and Dufresne 1996). A 1998 study comparing Israeli patients on clozapine ($n=30$) and typical antipsychotics ($n=30$) for at least 1 year confirmed the presence of hypertriglyceridemia in the clozapine group (202.9 mg/dL) but not the typical group (134.4 mg/dL), again without significant differences in total cholesterol (clozapine 197 mg/dL vs. typical 194.9 mg/dL) (Spivak et al. 1999). Yet a small retrospective study of clozapine patients ($n=19$) treated for 2 years found a 17.9% increase in total cholesterol, with a strong ($r=0.9$, $P=0.009$) correlation with serum LDL (Cato et al. 2000).

Olanzapine, another dibenzodiazepine compound, is also associated with significant elevations in serum triglyceride concentrations, with one case series documenting fasting serum levels in separate individuals of 2,061 mg/dL, 2,811 mg/dL, and 7,668 mg/dL (Meyer 2001b). In a 1-year study of chronic nongeriatric adult inpatients, the olanzapine group exhibited a mean increase in serum triglyceride concentration of 104.8 mg/dL compared with 31.7 mg/dL for the risperidone cohort (P=0.037), and a 30.4 mg/dL increase was seen in TC compared with only 7.2 mg/dL for the risperidone cohort (P=0.004) (Meyer 2002). One prospective study comparing risperidone and olanzapine in a group of males (n=22 each) showed 10.3% greater serum LDL after 17 months of therapy for the olanzapine cohort, but this was not significant at the 0.05 level; however, there was a trend (P=0.06) for higher TC to HDL ratio for the olanzapine group (Bouchard et al. 2001). Finally, prospective data presented from a large 6-week randomized study revealed a nonsignificant decrease in fasting LDL for the ziprasidone arm (n=106), whereas the olanzapine cohort (n=105) exhibited a significant 12.0% increase in fasting LDL (Glick et al. 2001). After adjusting for baseline differences, the serum LDL in the olanzapine cohort was 13.0% greater than in the ziprasidone group. Moreover, there was not a consistent finding in these and other studies that lipid elevations were closely correlated with dose or changes in weight. Ethnicity also appears not to be a factor, because both Caucasians and African Americans exposed to olanzapine experienced substantial increases in serum triglyceride concentrations (81% and 65%, respectively) (Nasrallah et al. 2001).

Both risperidone and ziprasidone are nondibenzodiazepine atypical antipsychotics and, as indicated here, appear to have minimal effects on serum lipids. Between these two compounds, ziprasidone is the more lipid neutral, with data from 6-week open-label studies of patients switched from olanzapine, risperidone, and typicals showing statistically significant decreases in median nonfasting TC and triglycerides (Daniel et al. 2000; Kingsbury et al. 2001). One short-term study (average treatment 15–25 days) associated ziprasidone and risperidone with decreases in fasting triglyceride concentration, although the magnitude of decrease was much greater for the ziprasidone cohort (P<0.05) (Pfizer 2000).

Limited data exist for quetiapine, yet as a dibenzothiazepine it appears to share a propensity for hyperlipidemia with its structural analogues. Among Meyer's case series of severe hypertriglyceridemia patients were two receiving quetiapine therapy, one of whom achieved a fasting triglyceride concentration of 1,911 mg/dL (Meyer 2001b). Quetiapine therapy was also associated with an elevated TC to HDL ratio compared with ziprasidone (P<0.01) in the short-term study noted previously (Pfizer 2000).

The effects of dibenzodiazepine-derived compounds on cardiovascular risk can be seen in Table 4–3, which presents data from a 26-year-old male state hospital patient treated with olanzapine. Utilizing the point scale from the risk chart in Table 4–2, one can see that the use of olanzapine quadrupled his risk for a major coronary event over the next decade. Moreover, if this patient had been 46 and not 26, the risk of a major coronary event would have increased 100%, giving him a 20% chance of a major coronary event in the next 10 years. It is worth noting that the peak serum triglyceride concentration in this patient occurred after 11 months of therapy (408 mg/dL), a characteristic clinical course observed when serum lipids are serially monitored after the onset of dibenzodiazepine treatment. Peak triglyceride levels typically occur within the first year of therapy during the course of dibenzodiazepine therapy, followed by a decrease and subsequent period of stabilization. Wide interindividual variation exists in both the timing of peak triglyceride levels and the magnitude of lipid elevations, and this has implications for monitoring of serum lipids during therapy with the dibenzodiazepine-derived agents (Meyer 2001a).

Other Cardiovascular Effects of Antipsychotics

For decades antipsychotics have been associated with certain short-term reversible side effects such as tachycardia and orthostasis, derived from the propensity of certain agents to antagonize muscarinic cholinergic and α_1-adrenergic receptors, respectively. The low-potency phenothiazine compounds, such as chlorpromazine and thioridazine, and the atypical antipsychotic clozapine are particularly noted for these side effects. Although resting tachycardia is often asymptomatic, and not treated until resting heart rates are consistently above 110 beats per minute, dizziness and falls related to orthostasis may be problematic, particularly for older patients who have poor vasomotor tone and possible postural instability related to parkinsonism or underlying central nervous system (CNS) pathology.

Prolongation of the Q–T interval (typically reported as QTc, corrected for heart rate) on electrocardiogram (ECG) is a cardiovascular side effect that has received significant attention due to the black-box warning placed in 2000 by the U.S. Food and Drug Administration (FDA) on thioridazine, mesoridazine, intramuscular droperidol, and pimozide because of this issue. Briefly, the concern arises from the fact that certain antipsychotics, by acting on myocardial potassium rectifier channels, delay repolarization, thereby increasing the QTc interval. Resting QTc is typically less than 420 ms for

Table 4–3. Effects of olanzapine on 10-year cardiovascular risk in a 26-year-old male

	Baseline			16 months of olanzapine		
	Values	Points	Points (if age 46)	Values	Points	Points (if age 47)
Age (years)	26	−9	3	27	−9	3
Smoking	Yes	8	5	Yes	8	5
Systolic blood pressure	125 mm Hg untreated	0	0	125 mm Hg untreated	0	0
Total cholesterol	174 mg/dL	4	3	238 mg/dL	7	5
HDL cholesterol	40 mg/dL	1	1	35 mg/dL	2	2
Triglyceride	168 mg/dL	N/A	N/A	339 mg/dL	N/A	N/A
Point totals		4	12		8	15
10-year cardiovascular risk		1%	10%		4% (↑300%)	20% (↑100%)

Note. HDL = high-density lipoprotein; N/A = not applicable.

males and 430 ms for females, with the risk for syncope or sudden death due to arrhythmia (torsades de pointes, ventricular fibrillation) increasing significantly for QTc greater than 500 ms. The drug manufacturer Pfizer was required to submit data to the FDA on this issue in July 2000 in support of their compound ziprasidone (Pfizer 2000). This report, known as the 054 Study, found thioridazine to have the greatest prolongation of QTc (35.6 ms at steady state), compared with haloperidol (4.7 ms); ziprasidone (20.3 ms); and risperidone, olanzapine, or quetiapine (all <15 ms). On the basis of these and other results, thioridazine and the other compounds mentioned above received a black-box warning mandating ECG monitoring during therapy; the product labeling for ziprasidone contains only boldface type concerning use in certain patient populations, with no ECG requirements. Prolongation of the QTc interval related to drug therapy is reversible on discontinuation of the offending agent, although one should bear in mind that drugs from various classes (e.g., diuretics, quinolone antibiotics) may cause this effect. (For further discussion of QTc prolongation related to drug therapy, see the concise review by Glassman and Bigger in the *American Journal of Psychiatry* [Glassman and Bigger 2001].)

Clinical Recommendations and Conclusions

Increasingly, psychiatrists and mental health clinics who treat the chronically mentally ill recognize that they have become de facto primary care providers for these patients, who often have limited access to outside medical services. Integrated medical and psychiatric care appears promising in achieving important health gains for patients with schizophrenia, yet is not the reality for most mental health settings (Druss et al. 2001). A certain amount of nihilism combined with the need to immediately focus on major psychopathology often leaves chronic medical issues unaddressed by mental health practitioners (Le Fevre 2001). Moreover, patients with schizophrenia do not adequately communicate their health problems and needs (Pary and Barton 1988). Nonetheless, data reveal improved compliance with medications and health recommendations after educational intervention (Kelly et al. 1990). Therefore, one should not eschew lifestyle counseling, as the benefits seen with even modest changes in cardiovascular risk factors are greatest in those with high cardiovascular risk.

At a minimum, improving cardiovascular risk and overall health starts with an awareness of the inherent vulnerability of patients with schizophrenia to cardiovascular disease, and the impetus to engage in screening for important risk factors (Braunstein et al. 2001). Interventions related to obesity, smoking, and DM or glucose intolerance are discussed at length in Chapters 2, 5, and 6 of this volume. Most of the basic screening for major cardiovascular risk factors can be accomplished in a few minutes, including asking questions about smoking status, family history of premature CHD (CHD in male first-degree relative <55 years old or female first-degree relative <65 years old), personal history of MI or angina, measurement of blood pressure and weight, and ordering the appropriate monitoring labs as discussed later. At present, there is not a general consensus for routine electrocardiographic monitoring in all patients as a tool for predicting long-term cardiovascular risk. Such risk is better assessed through evaluation of conventional cardiovascular risk factors, because studies demonstrate that the apparent low sensitivity of the ECG to future coronary events makes it impractical as a screening tool (Ashley et al. 2001).

Specific Lipid Monitoring Recommendations for Patients With Schizophrenia

Given the fact that patients with schizophrenia typically possess multiple cardiovascular risk factors, a full lipid panel with fractionation of cholesterol should be performed annually as part of routine health monitoring for inpatients and outpatients. With higher-risk agents for hyperlipidemia (clozapine, olanzapine, quetiapine), quarterly fasting triglycerides and TC can be considered for ongoing screening instead of the more expensive lipid panel during the first year of atypical antipsychotic therapy. This monitoring frequency for higher-risk agents is necessary to detect severe hypertriglyceridemia, which presents a risk for acute pancreatitis at triglyceride levels much greater than 500 mg/dL, and particularly at those above 1,000 mg/dL. After 1 year the monitoring frequency for patients on dibenzodiazepine-derived compounds may be decreased to annual assessment depending on the results. Although it is sometimes difficult to obtain reliable fasting specimens on outpatients, both TC and HDL are valid on nonfasting specimens.

On the basis of the laboratory and clinical data, one should calculate 10-year cardiovascular risk estimates and determine the need to refer patients for pharmacotherapy, including those with modest lipid abnormalities. (The National Heart, Lung and Blood Institute [NHLBI] has posted a useful summary of the recent NCEP guidelines for Palm operating system–based PDAs on its Web site: hin.nhlbi.nih.gov/atpiii/atp3palm.htm.) Diet and lifestyle modification are considered the mainstays of cardiovascular risk reduction, and counseling in these areas should always be offered;

however, when dietary measures have failed to normalize serum lipids, results from the landmark statin trials should make it abundantly clear that simple pharmacological interventions in those with low HDL, high LDL, or elevated triglycerides or TC may yield substantial reductions in cardiovascular morbidity and mortality. Nonetheless, undertreatment of hyperlipidemia is an ongoing problem for many patients, even those without major mental illness who have established CHD (Smith 2000). Although mental health practitioners may not choose to institute lipid agents themselves, patients with established CHD or CHD-equivalent disorders (e.g., DM, severe atherosclerotic vascular disease) should be started on low-dose aspirin therapy (81 mg/day, or one baby aspirin); this simple intervention has been proven to reduce important vascular events by 25%–33% (Braunstein et al. 2001). On the other hand, some psychiatrists may feel comfortable initiating treatment of hyperlipidemia under the guidance of an internist, cardiologist, or family practitioner because the typical first-line medications employed, statins and fibrates (e.g., fenofibrate, gemfibrozil), are relatively safe when used individually, although there is a necessity for occasional monitoring of liver function tests and creatine kinase.

In all instances, patients with schizophrenia and persistent hyperlipidemia must receive lipid-lowering therapy geared toward lipid goals defined by level of cardiovascular risk to minimize the likelihood of CHD and death from coronary disease. As mental health practitioners, it is important not to lose sight of the significant impact that nonpsychiatric medical comorbidity has on the chronically mentally ill. The dramatic reductions in coronary morbidity and mortality from hyperlipidemia treatment is one of the most powerful interventions available in medicine today, and this treatment should be widely available to patients with schizophrenia, who represent a group at high risk for cardiovascular disease.

References

Allison DB, Fontaine KR, Heo M, et al: The distribution of body mass index among individuals with and without schizophrenia. J Clin Psychiatry 60:215–220, 1999a

Allison DB, Mentore JL, Heo M, et al: Antipsychotic-induced weight gain: a comprehensive research synthesis. Am J Psychiatry 156:1686–1696, 1999b

Allison DB, Casey DE: Antipsychotic-induced weight gain: a review of the literature. J Clin Psychiatry 62 (suppl 7):22–31, 2001

Ascher-Svanum H, Tunis SL, Prudence L, et al: Prevalence of risk factors for coronary heart disease in schizophrenia. Poster presented at the American Psychiatric Association Annual Meeting, New Orleans, LA, May 8, 2001

Ashley EA, Raxwal V, Froelicher V: An evidence-based review of the resting electrocardiogram as a screening technique for heart disease. Prog Cardiovasc Dis 44:55–67, 2001

Bakx JC, van den Hoogen HJ, Deurenberg P, et al: Changes in serum total cholesterol levels over 18 years in a cohort of men and women: the Nijmegen Cohort Study. Prev Med 30:138–145, 2000

Bakx JC, Veldstra MI, van den Hoogen HM, et al: Blood pressure and cardiovascular morbidity and mortality in a Dutch population: the Nijmegen cohort study. Prev Med 32:142–147, 2001

Bard JM, Charles MA, Juhan-Vague I, et al: Accumulation of triglyceride-rich lipoprotein in subjects with abdominal obesity: the Biguanides and the Prevention of the Risk of Obesity (BIGPRO) 1 Study. Arterioscler Thromb Vasc Biol 21:407–414, 2001

Bellnier TJ, Labrum AH, Patil KB, et al: Prevalence of cardiovascular disease comorbidities and risk factors in severe and persistently mentally ill patients. Poster presented at the American Psychiatric Association Annual Meeting, New Orleans, LA, May 8, 2001

Blackburn GL: Weight gain and antipsychotic medication. J Clin Psychiatry 61 (suppl 8):36–41, 2000

Bouchard RH, Demers M-F, Simoneau I, et al: Atypical antipsychotics and cardiovascular risk in schizophrenic patients. J Clin Psychopharmacol 21:110–111, 2001

Braun GA and Paulonis ME: Sterol metabolism: biochemical differences among the butyrophenones. Int J Neuropsychiatry 3 (suppl):26–27, 1967

Braunstein JB, Cheng A, Fakhry C, et al: ABCs of cardiovascular disease risk management. Cardiol Rev 9:96–105, 2001

Brown S, Birtwistle J, Roe L, et al: The unhealthy lifestyle of people with schizophrenia. Psychol Med 29:697–701, 1999

Brown S, Inskip H, Barraclough B: Causes of the excess mortality of schizophrenia. Br J Psychiatry 177:212–217, 2000

Casey DE: Prevalence of diabetes during extended clozapine and olanzapine treatment. Poster presented at the American College of Neuropsychopharmacology Annual Meeting, San Juan, Puerto Rico, December 10–14, 2000

Cato MM, Yovtcheva SP, Stanley-Tilt CA, et al: Metabolic and cardiovascular consequences of prolonged clozapine treatment: a retrospective study. Poster presented at the American Psychiatric Association Annual Meeting, Chicago, IL, May 15, 2000

Chute D, Grove C, Rajasekhara B, et al: Schizophrenia and sudden death: a medical examiner case study. Am J Forensic Med Pathol 20:131–135, 1999

Clark ML, Ray TS, Paredes A, et al: Chlorpromazine in women with chronic schizophrenia: the effect on cholesterol levels and cholesterol-behavior relationships. Psychosom Med 29:634–642, 1967

Coffman JA, Olshansky B, Nasrallah HA, et al: Echocardiographic assessment of schizophrenics and manics: a reexamination of early necropsy findings. J Nerv Ment Dis 173:179–181, 1985

Cohn T, Remington G: Risk factors for coronary vascular disease in long-term psychiatric inpatients on typical and atypical antipsychotic medications. Paper presented at the International Congress on Schizophrenia Research, Whistler, BC, Canada, April 30, 2001

Coutinho M, Gerstein HC, Wang Y, et al: The relationship between glucose and incident cardiovascular events: a metaregression analysis of published data from 20 studies of 95,783 individuals followed for 12.4 years. Diabetes Care 22:233–240, 1999

Cullen P: Evidence that triglycerides are an independent coronary heart disease risk factor. Am J Cardiol 86:943–949, 2000

Curkendall SM, Mo J, Jones JK, et al: Increased cardiovascular disease in patients with schizophrenia. Poster presented at the annual meeting of the American Psychiatric Association, New Orleans, LA, May 8, 2001

Daniel DG, Weiden P, O'Sullivan RL: Improvements in indices of health status in outpatients with schizophrenia following a switch to ziprasidone from conventional antipsychotics, olanzapine or risperidone. Poster presented at the annual meeting of the American Psychiatric Association, Chicago, IL, May 15, 2000

Davidson S, Judd F, Jolley D, et al: Cardiovascular risk factors for people with mental illness. Aust N Z J Psychiatry 35:196–202, 2001

de Leon J, Dadvand M, Canuso C, et al: Schizophrenia and smoking: an epidemiological survey in a state hospital. Am J Psychiatry 152:453–455, 1995

Dixon L, Postrado L, Delahanty J, et al: The association of medical comorbidity in schizophrenia with poor physical and mental health. J Nerv Ment Dis 187:496–502, 1999

Dixon L, Weiden P, Delahanty J, et al: Prevalence and correlates of diabetes in national schizophrenia samples. Schizophr Bull 26:903–912, 2000

Downs JR, Clearfield M, Weis S, et al: Primary prevention of acute coronary events with lovastatin in men and women with average cholesterol levels: results of the Air Force/Texas Coronary Atherosclerosis Prevention Study. JAMA 279:1615–1622, 1998

Druss BG, Bradford DW, Rosenheck RA, et al: Mental disorders and use of cardiovascular procedures after myocardial infarction. JAMA 283:506–511, 2000

Druss B, Rohrbaugh RM, Levinson CM, et al: Integrated medical care for patients with serious psychiatric illness: a randomized trial. Arch Gen Psychiatry 58:861–868, 2001

Eder U, Mangweth B, Ebenbichler C, et al: Association of olanzapine-induced weight gain with an increase in body fat. Am J Psychiatry 158:1719–1722, 2001

Eliasson B, Hjalmarson A, Kruse E, et al: Effect of smoking reduction and cessation on cardiovascular risk factors. Nicotine Tob Res 3:249–255, 2001

Engstrom G, Berglund G, Goransson M, et al: Distribution and determinants of ischaemic heart disease in an urban population: a study from the myocardial infarction register in Malmo, Sweden. J Intern Med 247:588–596, 2000

Expert Panel on Detection, Evaluation, and Treatment of High Blood Cholesterol in Adults: Executive summary of the third report of the National Cholesterol Education Program (NCEP) Expert Panel on Detection, Evaluation, and Treatment of High Blood Cholesterol in Adults (Adult Treatment Panel III). JAMA 285:2486–2497, 2001

Flegal KM, Troiano RP: Changes in the distribution of body mass index of adults and children in the US population. Int J Obes Relat Metab Disord 24:807–818, 2000

Fleischhacker WW, Stuppack C, Moser C, et al: Fluperlapine vs haloperidol: a comparison of their neuroendocrinological profiles and the influence on serum lipids. Pharmacopsychiatry 19:111–114, 1986

Ford ES, Giles WH, Dietz WH: Prevalence of the metabolic syndrome among US adults: findings from the third National Health and Nutrition Examination Survey. JAMA 287:356–359, 2002

Gerstein HC, Pais P, Pogue J, et al: Relationship of glucose and insulin levels to the risk of myocardial infarction: a case-control study. J Am Coll Cardiol 33:612–619, 1999

Gerstein HC, Mann JF, Yi Q, et al: Albuminuria and risk of cardiovascular events, death, and heart failure in diabetic and nondiabetic individuals. JAMA 286:421–426, 2001

Ghaeli P, Dufresne RL: Serum triglyceride levels in patients treated with clozapine. Am J Health Syst Pharm 53:2079–2081, 1996

Glassman AH, Bigger JT: Antipsychotic drugs: prolonged QTc interval, torsade de pointes, and sudden death. Am J Psychiatry 158:1774–1782, 2001

Glick ID, Romano SJ, Simpson GM, et al: Insulin resistance in olanzapine- and ziprasidone-treated patients: results of a double-blind, controlled 6-week trial. Poster presented at the annual meeting of the American Psychiatric Association, New Orleans, LA, May 8, 2001

Grundy SM: Hypertriglyceridemia, insulin resistance, and the metabolic syndrome. Am J Cardiol 83:25F–29F, 1999

Haupt DW, Newcomer JW, Fucetola R, et al: Glucose regulation during antipsychotic treatment in schizophrenia. Poster presented at the American Association of Geriatric Psychiatrists, San Francisco, CA, February 23–26, 2001

Henderson DC, Cagliero E, Gray C, et al: Clozapine, diabetes mellitus, weight gain, and lipid abnormalities: a five-year naturalistic study. Am J Psychiatry 157:975–981, 2000

Hoerger TJ, Bala MV, Bray JW, et al: Treatment patterns and distribution of low-density lipoprotein cholesterol levels in treatment-eligible United States adults. Am J Cardiol 82:61–65, 1998

Hooper L, Summerbell CD, Higgins JP, et al: Dietary fat intake and prevention of cardiovascular disease: systematic review. BMJ 322:757–763, 2001

Hughes JR, Hatsukami DK, Mitchell JE, et al: Prevalence of smoking among psychiatric outpatients. Am J Psychiatry 143:993–997, 1986

Jeppesen J, Hein HO, Suadicani P, et al: Triglyceride concentration and ischemic heart disease: an eight-year follow-up in the Copenhagen Male Study. Circulation 97:1029–1036, 1998

Jones AF, Walker J, Jewkes C, et al: Comparative accuracy of cardiovascular risk prediction methods in primary care patients. Heart 85:37–43, 2001

Kelly C, McCreadie RG: Smoking habits, current symptoms, and premorbid characteristics of schizophrenic patients in Nithsdale, Scotland. Am J Psychiatry 156:1751–1756, 1999

Kelly GR, Scott JE, Mamon J: Medication compliance and health education among outpatients with chronic mental disorders. Med Care 28:1181–1197, 1990

Kingsbury SJ, Fayek M, Trufasiu D, et al: The apparent effects of ziprasidone on plasma lipids and glucose. J Clin Psychiatry 62:347–349, 2001

Kohl HW III: Physical activity and cardiovascular disease: evidence for a dose-response. Med Sci Sports Exerc 33 (suppl 6):S472–S483, S493–S494, 2001

Kromhout D: Diet and cardiovascular diseases. J Nutr Health Aging 5:144–149, 2001

Kwiterovich PO Jr: The metabolic pathways of high-density lipoprotein, low-density lipoprotein, and triglycerides: a current review. Am J Cardiol 86:5L–10L, 2000

Law MR, Morris JK, Wald NJ: Environmental tobacco smoke exposure and ischaemic heart disease: an evaluation of the evidence. BMJ 315:973–980, 1997

Le Fevre PD: Improving the physical health of patients with schizophrenia: therapeutic nihilism or realism? Scott Med J 46:11–31, 2001

Lee IM, Skerrett PJ: Physical activity and all-cause mortality: what is the dose-response relation? Med Sci Sports Exerc 33(suppl 6):S459–S471, 2001

Liese AD, Hense HW, Brenner H, et al: Assessing the impact of classical risk factors on myocardial infarction by rate advancement periods. Am J Epidemiol 152:884–888, 2000

LIPID Sutdy Group: Prevention of cardiovascular events and death with pravastatin in patients with coronary heart disease and a broad range of initial cholesterol levels: the Long-Term Intervention with Pravastatin in Ischaemic Disease (LIPID) Study Group. N Engl J Med 339:1349–1357, 1998

Mantel-Teeuwisse AK, Kloosterman JM, Maitland-van der Zee AH, et al: Drug-induced lipid changes: a review of the unintended effects of some commonly used drugs on serum lipid levels. Drug Saf 24:443–456, 2001

Marques-Vidal P, Montaye M, Haas B, et al: Relationships between alcoholic beverages and cardiovascular risk factor levels in middle-aged men: the PRIME Study—Prospective Epidemiological Study of Myocardial Infarction Study. Atherosclerosis 157:431–440, 2001

McCarron DA, Reusser ME: The power of food to improve multiple cardiovascular risk factors. Curr Atheroscler Rep 2:482–486, 2000

McIntyre RS, McCann SM, Kennedy SH: Antipsychotic metabolic effects: weight gain, diabetes mellitus, and lipid abnormalities. Can J Psychol 46:273–281, 2001

Mefferd RB, Labrosse EH, Gawienowski AM, et al: Influence of chlorpromazine on certain biochemical variables of chronic male schizophrenics. J Nerv Ment Dis 127:167–179, 1958

Melanson KJ, McInnis KJ, Rippe JM, et al: Obesity and cardiovascular disease risk: research update. Cardiol Rev 9:202–207, 2001

Meyer JM: Effects of atypical antipsychotics on weight and serum lipids. J Clin Psychiatry 62 (suppl 27):27–34, 2001a

Meyer JM: Novel antipsychotics and severe hyperlipidemia. J Clin Psychopharmacol 21:369–374, 2001b

Meyer JM: A retrospective comparison of lipid, glucose and weight changes at one year between olanzapine and risperidone treated inpatients. J Clin Psychiatry 63:425–433, 2002

Millen BE, Quatromoni PA: Nutritional research within the Framingham Heart Study. J Nutr Health Aging 5:139–143, 2001

Muller-Oerlinghausen B: A short survey on untoward effects of fluperlapine. Arzneimittelforschung 34:131–134, 1984

Nasrallah HA, Perry CL, Love E, et al: Are there ethnic differences in hypertriglyceridemia secondary to olanzapine treatment? Poster presented at the 40th annual meeting of the American College of Neuropsychopharmacology, Waikoloa, HI, December 2001

Olincy A, Young DA, Freedman R: Increased levels of the nicotine metabolite cotinine in schizophrenic smokers compared to other smokers. Biol Psychiatry 42:1–5, 1997

Osby U, Correia N, Brandt L, et al: Mortality and causes of death in schizophrenia in Stockholm County, Sweden. Schizophr Res 45:21–28, 2000

Pary RJ, Barton, SN: Communication difficulty of patients with schizophrenia and physical illness. South Med J 81:489–490, 1988

Pearson TA: The undertreatment of LDL-cholesterol: addressing the challenge. Int J Cardiol 74 (suppl 1):S23–S28, 2000

Pearson TA, Boden WE: The imperative to raise low levels of high-density lipoprotein in cholesterol: a better clinical strategy in the prevention and treatment of coronary artery disease—introduction. Am J Cardiol 86:1L–4L, 2000

Pereira MA, Pins JJ: Dietary fiber and cardiovascular disease: experimental and epidemiologic advances. Curr Atheroscler Rep 2:494–502, 2000

Perreault S, Dorais M, Coupal L, et al: Impact of treating hyperlipidemia or hypertension to reduce the risk of death from coronary artery disease. CMAJ 160:1449–1455, 1999

Pfizer: Briefing document for ziprasidone HCl presented at the FDA Psychopharmacological Drugs Advisory Committee July 19, 2000

Pietinen P, Lahti-Koski M, Vertiainen E, et al: Nutrition and cardiovascular disease in Finland since the early 1970s: a success story. J Nutr Health Aging 5:150–154, 2001

Rossner S, Sjostrom L, Noack R, et al: Weight loss, weight maintenance, and improved cardiovascular risk factors after 2 years treatment with orlistat for obesity: European Orlistat Obesity Study Group. Obes Res 8:49–61, 2000

Rubins HB: Triglycerides and coronary heart disease: implications of recent clinical trials. J Cardiovasc Risk 7:339–345, 2000

Ruschena D, Mullen PE, Burgess P, et al: Sudden death in psychiatric patients. Br J Psychiatry 172:331–336, 1998

Sacks FM, Pfeffer MA, Moye LA, et al: The effect of pravastatin on coronary events after myocardial infarction in patients with average cholesterol levels: Cholesterol and Recurrent Events Trial investigators. N Engl J Med 335:1001–1009, 1996

Sasaki J, Kumagae G, Sata T, et al: Decreased concentration of high density lipoprotein cholesterol in schizophrenic patients treated with phenothiazines. Atherosclerosis 51:163–169, 1984

Sasaki J, Funakoshi M, Arakawa K: Lipids and apolipoproteins in patients treated with major tranquilizers. Clin Pharmacol Ther 37:684–687, 1985

Scandinavian Simvastatin Survival Study (4S): Randomised trial of cholesterol lowering in 4444 patients with coronary heart disease: the Scandinavian Simvastatin Survival Study (4S). Lancet 344:1383–1389, 1994

Shepherd J, Cobbe SM, Ford I, et al: Prevention of coronary heart disease with pravastatin in men with hypercholesterolemia: West of Scotland Coronary Prevention Study Group. N Engl J Med 333:1301–1307, 1995

Simpson GM, Cooper TB: The effect of three butyrophenones on serum cholesterol levels. Curr Ther Res 8:249–255, 1966

Simpson GM, Cooper TB, Braun GA: Further studies on the effect of butyrophenones on cholesterol synthesis in humans. Curr Ther Res 9:413–418, 1967

Smith CJ, Fischer TH, Sears SB: Environmental tobacco smoke, cardiovascular disease, and the nonlinear dose-response hypothesis. Toxicol Sci 54:462–472, 2000

Smith SC Jr: Clinical treatment of dyslipidemia: practice patterns and missed opportunities. Am J Cardiol 86:62L–65L, 2000

Spivak B, Lamschtein C, Talmon Y, et al: The impact of clozapine treatment on serum lipids in chronic schizophrenic patients. Clin Neuropharmacol 22:98–101, 1999

Stamler J, Wentworth D, Neaton JD: Is relationship between serum cholesterol and risk of premature death from coronary heart disease continuous and graded? Findings in 356,222 primary screenees of the Multiple Risk Factor Intervention Trial (MRFIT). JAMA 256:2823–2828, 1986

Strandberg TE, Salomaa VV, Vanhanen HT, et al: Blood pressure and mortality during an up to 32-year follow-up. J Hypertens 19:35–39, 2001

Villablanca AC, McDonald JM, Rutledge JC: Smoking and cardiovascular disease. Clin Chest Med 21:159–172, 2000

Wannamethee SG, Shaper AG: Physical activity in the prevention of cardiovascular disease: an epidemiological perspective. Sports Med 31:101–114, 2001

Wilson PW, Abbott RD, Castelli WP: High density lipoprotein cholesterol and mortality: the Framingham Heart Study. Arteriosclerosis 8:737–741, 1988

Wood D, Joint European Societies Task Force: Established and emerging cardiovascular risk factors. Am Heart J 141 (suppl 2):S49–S57, 2001

Chapter 5

Nicotine and Tobacco Use in Schizophrenia

Tony P. George, M.D.
Jennifer C. Vessicchio, M.S.W.
Angelo Termine, B.S.

Epidemiology and Significance of the Problem

Several epidemiological and clinical studies since the 1980s have documented the high rates of cigarette smoking in psychiatric patients, particularly those with schizophrenia-related disorders (Chong and Choo 1996; de Leon et al. 1995; Diwan et al. 1998; el-Guebaly and Hodgins 1992; George et al. 1995; Goff et al. 1992; Hughes et al. 1986; Kelly and McCredie 1999; Masterson and O'Shea 1984; McEvoy and Brown 1999; Menza et al. 1991; O'Farrell et al. 1983; Ziedonis et al. 1994).

This work was supported in part by grants R01-DA-13672, R01-DA-14039, and K12-DA-00167 to Dr. George from the National Institute on Drug Abuse (NIDA), and a Wodecroft Young Investigator Award to Dr. George from the National Alliance for Research on Schizophrenia and Depression (NARSAD).

Although smoking rates in the general population have substantially declined from 45% in the 1960s to about 25% currently (Vocci and DeWit 1999), rates of smoking in chronic psychiatric patients, especially those with schizophrenia, continue to be very high. In fact, one recent community-based study suggested that nearly 45% of all cigarette consumption in the United States is by individuals with mental disorders (Lasser et al. 2000). Surveys of cigarette smoking in schizophrenia in a myriad of inpatient and outpatient settings in several nations have found prevalence rates of 32%–92% (Table 5–1), with the variability in smoking rates attributable to such factors as disease chronicity, smoking accessibility, and social prohibitions on smoking behavior. What is not clear from these studies is the proportion of outpatient schizophrenic smokers that meet DSM-IV-TR criteria (American Psychiatric Association 2000) for nicotine dependence, because most studies have been conducted in treatment settings in which the likelihood of nicotine dependence is higher, whereas there is a paucity of data from structured surveys in community samples.

Although such dependence data are lacking, the generally high smoking prevalence noted in schizophrenia and other psychiatric populations may relate to an increased vulnerability to tobacco use and inability to achieve smoking cessation. This is particularly concerning because rates of smoking-related illnesses such as cardiovascular disease and certain cancers appear to be higher in patients with schizophrenia than in the general population (Lichtermann et al. 2001). Hence, there is an urgent need to address tobacco addiction in this population through the development of effective treatments, both pharmacological and psychosocial. A better understanding of the biology of tobacco addiction in schizophrenic patients may assist in the development of better treatments for tobacco use in this vulnerable population.

Pharmacology of Nicotine and Tobacco: Relevance to Schizophrenia

There has been an increasing understanding of the neurobiology of both schizophrenia and nicotine addiction in the past 20 years. For the purposes of this discussion, nicotine is assumed to be the active ingredient in tobacco and cigarette smoking that exerts psychopharmacological effects, though other components of tobacco smoke may also be active in this respect (Fowler et al. 1996a, 1996b). There are three possible reasons for the high comorbidity rates of nicotine addiction in schizophrenia: 1) self-medication of clinical and cognitive deficits associated with schizophrenia by tobacco use, 2) abnormalities in brain reward pathways in schizophrenia that make these patients

Table 5–1. Prevalence of cigarette smoking in individuals with schizophrenia

Study	Patient population	Smoking prevalence rate (%)
O'Farrell et al. (1983)	309 veteran inpatients in United States	88 (*n*=207 schizophrenic patients)
Masterson and O'Shea (1984)	100 schizophrenic inpatients in Ireland	83 (84% in males, 82% in females)
Hughes et al. (1986)	277 psychiatric outpatients in United States	88 (*n*=24 schizophrenic patients)
el-Guebaly and Hodgins (1992)	106 schizophrenic inpatients in Canada	61
Menza et al. (1991)	126 psychiatric outpatients in United States	56 (*n*=99 schizophrenic patients)
Goff et al. (1992)	78 schizophrenic outpatients in United States	74
Ziedonis et al. (1994)	265 schizophrenic outpatients in United States	68
de Leon et al. (1995)	237 schizophrenic inpatients in United States	85
George et al. (1995)	29 schizophrenic outpatients on clozapine in United States	62.1
Chong and Chou (1996)	195 schizophrenic outpatients in China	31.8 (control rate 16%)
Diwan et al. (1998)	63 schizophrenic veteran outpatients in United States	86
McEvoy and Brown (1999)	12 first-episode schizophrenic patients in United States	92
Kelly and McCredie (1999)	168 schizophrenic outpatients in Scotland	58
	Composite smoking prevalence	**72.5**

vulnerable to tobacco (and other drug) use, and 3) common genetic and environmental factors that are independently associated with smoking and schizophrenia. We briefly describe next the pharmacological effects of nicotine and how such effects may link nicotine addiction with schizophrenia.

Nicotine alters the function of neurotransmitter systems implicated in the pathogenesis of major psychiatric disorders, including dopamine, norepinephrine, serotonin (5-HT), glutamate, gamma-aminobutyric acid (GABA), and endogenous opioid peptides (George et al. 2000b, 2000c; McGehee et al. 1995; Picciotto et al. 2000). Nicotine's receptor in the brain is the nicotinic acetylcholine receptor (nAChR), where stimulation of presynaptic nAChRs on neurons increases transmitter release and metabolism. Unlike most agonists, chronic nicotine administration leads to desensitization and inactivation of nAChRs (Collins et al. 1994; Picciotto et al. 2000), with subsequent upregulation of nAChR sites, a process that might explain why many smokers report that the most satisfying cigarette of the day is the first one in the morning. Mesolimbic dopamine (reward pathway) neurons possess presynaptic nAChRs and may be of particular importance in mediating the rewarding effects of nicotine through projections from the ventral tegmental area (VTA) in the midbrain to anterior forebrain structures such as the nucleus accumbens and cingulate cortex. These are the same subcortical dopamine pathways that are implicated in the expression of the positive symptoms of schizophrenia. Similarly, there are nAChRs present presynaptically on midbrain dopamine neurons that project from the VTA to the prefrontal cortex (PFC) that evoke dopamine release and metabolism when activated by nicotine (during smoking). Dysregulation of PFC functioning has been demonstrated in schizophrenia, a finding possibly related to hypofunction of cortical dopamine and other transmitter systems (Knable and Weinberger 1997). It is this hypofunction of PFC dopamine that is thought to mediate the cognitive deficits and negative symptoms associated with schizophrenia and that may be ameliorated by cigarette smoking (George et al. 2000a, 2002a). Nicotine also stimulates glutamate release (McGehee et al. 1995) and could thereby alter abnormalities in central glutamatergic systems (e.g., hypofunction) associated with schizophrenia (Dalack et al. 1998).

Pharmacokinetic Implications of Smoking for Psychotropic Drug Use in Schizophrenia

There is strong evidence that tobacco smoking produces induction of the cytochrome P450 (CYP) 1A2 enzyme system in the liver, a major route for the metabolism of antipsychotic drugs such as haloperidol, chlorpromazine, olanzapine, and clozapine (George and Vessicchio 2001; Perry et al. 1993). Accordingly, smoking cessation may be expected to lead to increases in plasma concentrations of antipsychotic drugs metabolized by the 1A2 system, a finding demonstrated in both prospective and retrospective studies using both between-subject (Perry et al. 1993, 1998; Seppala et al. 1999) and within-subject (Meyer 2001) designs. Such an increase in circulating levels would be expected to increase the likelihood of extrapyramidal reactions and other antipsychotic drug side effects. A nomogram has been developed for clozapine in an attempt to aid clinicians in adjusting clozapine doses in smoking compared with nonsmoking schizophrenic subjects (Perry et al. 1998). Although no smoking cessation study in schizophrenics to date has prospectively measured antipsychotic plasma levels before and after smoking cessation, Meyer (2001) reported on serial clozapine levels measured in 11 patients with schizophrenia or schizoaffective disorder treated with stable doses in a state hospital before and after a hospital-wide ban on smoking. A mean increase of 57.4% was noted in these clozapine-treated patients who quit smoking; one patient in particular had an increase in his serum clozapine level to over 3,000 ng/mL that was associated with aspiration. In the few published controlled smoking cessation trials in this population (Addington 1998; George et al. 2000a, 2002b), no significant increases in medication side effects were noted in patients who quit smoking, including those treated with medications known to be metabolized by CYP 1A2, but further study is clearly warranted.

Effects of Nicotine and Smoking on Clinical and Cognitive Deficits Associated With Schizophrenia

Several cross-sectional studies have examined the effects of cigarette smoking on psychotic symptoms in schizophrenic patients (Goff et al. 1992; Hall et al. 1995; Ziedonis et al. 1994). Goff and colleagues found that schizophrenic smokers had higher Brief Psychiatric Rating Scale (BPRS) total scores than schizophrenic nonsmokers, and higher subscale scores for both positive and negative symptoms. Ziedonis and colleagues found increased positive symptom scores and reduced negative symptom scores in smoking versus nonsmoking schizophrenic patients, with heavy smokers having the highest positive and lowest negative symptom scores. Hall and colleagues noted that schizophrenic patients who were former smokers had fewer negative symptoms than current schizophrenic smokers, yet a recent study by our group found that schizophrenic former smokers had more negative symptoms than current smokers after adjustment for differences in age, depressive symptoms, and education (George et al. 2002a). Interestingly, one report suggested that smoking was reduced in schizophrenic patients reporting an exacerbation of psychotic symptoms (Hamera et al. 1995), whereas Dalack and colleagues (Dalack and Meador-Woodruff 1996) observed exacerbation of positive symptoms during smoking cessation or reduction.

There have been few direct studies of the effects of smoking or nicotine administration on clinical symptoms in patients with schizophrenia. In contrast to results from cross-sectional studies, controlled laboratory studies of smoking abstinence (Dalack et al. 1999; George et al. 2002a) and nicotine patch administration (Dalack and Meador-Woodruff 1999) have not shown significant effects on these clinical symptoms of schizophrenia. Furthermore, two recent smoking cessation trials (Addington et al. 1998; George et al. 2000a), in which all subjects used the nicotine patch, found no evidence of significant changes in psychotic symptoms with smoking abstinence in schizophrenic patients. Thus, the effects of cigarette smoking and smoking abstinence on schizophrenia symptoms are not clear. There may be some trait differences in psychotic symptoms in schizophrenic smokers versus nonsmokers (e.g., more refractory symptoms in nonsmokers) that could explain these findings, independent of smoking status (George et al. 2002a).

Cigarette smoking has been reported to reduce neuroleptic-induced parkinsonism (Decina et al. 1990; Goff et al. 1992; Sandyk 1993; Ziedonis et al. 1994), and may worsen symptoms of tardive dyskinesia (Yassa et al. 1987), but these effects have not been observed consistently in other studies (Dalack et al. 1998; Goff et al. 1992; Menza et al. 1991). Those properties leading to reduction in extrapyramidal side effects may relate to nicotine's enhancement of subcortical dopamine systems, but other transmitter systems, such as GABA and glutamate, are likely involved (Dalack et al. 1998).

Several human laboratory studies have suggested that schizophrenic subjects possess deficits in auditory information processing (P50 event-related potentials), which can be transiently normalized by cigarette smoking or administration of nicotine gum (Adler et al. 1993, 1998). In addition, these deficits in P50 responses in schizophrenics are improved by treatment with the atypical agent clozapine (Nagamoto et al. 1996) and other atypical antipsychotic agents (Light et al. 2000). Recent evidence has suggested that these P50 response deficits may be linked to a locus on chromosome 15 (q14) near the coding region for the α_7 nAChR (Freedman et al. 1997). This subtype of nAChR has been strongly implicated in

P50 responses, leading to speculation that if some schizophrenic patients possess defective α_7 nAChR–mediated neurotransmission, they may smoke heavily to overcome the related neurophysiological deficits. In addition, schizophrenic patients have abnormalities in another auditory information–processing response known as prepulse inhibition (PPI) of the acoustic startle reflex (Parwani et al. 2000; Swerdlow et al. 1992). The neural substrates mediating this response appear to be distinct from those mediating P50 responses (Swerdlow et al. 1992), and a recent study found that clozapine, but not typical antipsychotic drugs, appears to normalize deficits in PPI in schizophrenic patients (Kumari et al. 1999). Cigarette smoking may improve PPI, whereas acute smoking abstinence may impair it (George et al. 2001; Kumari et al. 1996). Thus, schizophrenic patients may be using cigarette smoking to ameliorate defects in cognitive function, further supporting the self-medication hypothesis of cigarette smoking in schizophrenia. This assertion is supported by 1) studies by Levin and colleagues demonstrating that the nicotine patch could dose-dependently reverse cognitive deficits associated with haloperidol administration in persons with schizophrenia (Levin et al. 1996) and 2) recent data on the effects of smoking abstinence on cognitive function in schizophrenic versus control smokers (George et al. 2002a).

The Yale Program for Research in Smokers with Mental Illness has studied cognitive function in schizophrenic and nonpsychiatric control subjects as a function of smoking status (George et al. 2002a). Although schizophrenic subjects compared with control subjects had deficits in visuospatial working memory (VSWM) function, a task dependent in part on prefrontal cortical dopamine function (Williams and Goldman-Rakic 1995), smoking appeared to improve these deficits in schizophrenic subjects and impair them in control subjects after adjustment for differences in age, educational attainment, and depressive symptoms between the four comparison groups. However, when schizophrenic smokers quit smoking during the course of a 10-week smoking cessation trial using bupropion hydrochloride (or placebo), deficits in VSWM were further impaired to the level of deficit in schizophrenic nonsmokers. In contrast, healthy control smokers who quit smoking in a smoking cessation trial with selegiline hydrochloride or placebo demonstrated improvements in VSWM function. These abstinence-induced changes in VSWM in both schizophrenic and control smokers appeared to be independent of the study medications used to facilitate smoking cessation (George et al. 2002a).

These preliminary results in schizophrenic versus control smokers, coupled with data on the effects of nicotine on the cortical dopamine system in animal studies (George et al. 1998, 2000c), allow one to propose a model

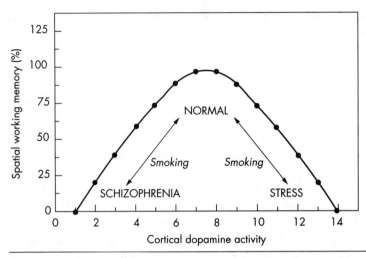

Figure 5–1. Relationship between cortical dopamine function and spatial working memory: effects of schizophrenia and cigarette smoking.

to explain the relationship between nicotine/smoking, cortical dopamine (and norepinephrine) function, and spatial working memory (Figure 5–1) (George et al. 1998, 2000b; Williams and Goldman-Rakic 1995).

Normal cortical dopamine function is associated with optimal levels of VSWM performance (Arnsten 2000; Williams and Goldman-Rakic 1995; Zahrt et al. 1997). In schizophrenic patients who have cortical dopamine hypofunction, VSWM is impaired, and nicotine administration through cigarette smoking leads to increases in cortical dopamine and improvements in VSWM (see Figure 5–1, Schizophrenia → Normal), whereas abstinence in the schizophrenic smoker impairs (Normal → Schizophrenia) VSWM, presumably in association with reductions in cortical dopamine activity as discussed previously. In control smokers, excessive cortical dopamine stimulation by cigarette smoking (see Figure 5–1, Normal → Stress) impairs VSWM (Park et al. 2000), similar to the effects of acute stress (George et al. 1998), and smoking abstinence in control subjects improves VSWM (Stress → Normal). Hence, the results from the Yale group are consistent with previous models that postulate an "inverted-U" relationship between cortical dopamine and spatial working memory, which is likely mediated by postsynaptic D_1 dopamine receptor stimulation (Arnsten 2000; Williams and Goldman-Rakic 1995; Zahrt et al. 1997). That is, too little (e.g., schizophrenia) or too much (e.g., produced by stress or smoking) cortical dopamine function impairs spatial working memory, and moderate levels of cortical dopamine activity are required for optimal spatial working memory function. In schizophrenic subjects, cigarette smoking (nicotine) augments VSWM (and cortical dopamine), and in control smokers, cigarette smoking impairs VSWM by producing cortical dopamine hyperfunction. This model may thus have important implications for the development of treatments for schizophrenia, and for nicotine addiction in these patients, possibly with the use of nonaddictive nicotinic receptor agonists.

Effects of Atypical Versus Typical Antipsychotic Drugs on Smoking in Schizophrenia

As reviewed previously, the Yale Program for Research in Smokers with Mental Illness group has found that switching schizophrenic smokers from typical antipsychotic agents to clozapine leads to reductions in self-reported cigarette smoking, especially in heavier smokers (George et al. 1995). Similar findings were reported by McEvoy et al., who found that the degree of reduction may be dependent on clozapine plasma levels (McEvoy et al. 1995a; McEvoy et al. 1999). A related study found that the typical antipsychotic drug haloperidol led to increased smoking in schizophrenic subjects compared with a baseline medication-free condition (McEvoy et al. 1995b). Thus, a role for atypical antipsychotic drugs in reducing smoking behavior is suggested.

Use of the nicotine transdermal patch (NTP) is known to facilitate smoking reduction (Dalack 1999) and cessation (Addington et al. 1998; George et al. 2000a) in schizophrenic smokers, albeit at lower rates (36%–42% at trial endpoint) than in healthy control smokers (50%–70%) (Balfour and Fagerstrom 1996). Nonetheless, NTP use at the dose of 21 mg/day appears to effectively reduce cigarette smoking and nicotine withdrawal symptoms in schizophrenic smokers (Addington et al. 1998; Dalack and Meador-Woodruff 1999; Dalack et al. 1999; George et al. 2000a). Other recent studies indicate that atypical antipsychotic drugs, in particular risperidone and olanzapine, may improve smoking cessation rates compared with typical antipsychotic drugs, in combination with the NTP, in schizophrenic smokers who had high motivation to quit smoking when they began the study (George et al. 2000a). Recent data from a preliminary placebo-controlled trial comparing bupropion versus placebo in schizophrenic smokers suggests that atypical antipsychotic treatment significantly enhances smoking cessation response to bupropion (George et al. 2002b).

One can speculate that atypical antipsychotic drugs may be helpful for smoking cessation in people with schizophrenia compared with typical neuroleptic agents for the following reasons: 1) atypical agents have fewer extrapyramidal side effects and improve negative symptoms, results that may also be achieved by cigarette smoking; 2) treatment with atypical agents is associated with improvement in certain neuropsychological functional deficits that also appear to be alleviated by smoking; 3) sensory gating deficits (e.g., P50 responses, prepulse inhibition) that are transiently normalized by nicotine administration or cigarette smoking are also ameliorated by atypical antipsychotic drugs (Light et al. 2000; Nagamoto et al. 1996); and 4) atypical agents are associated with augmentation of dopamine release in the prefrontal cortex in rodent studies (Ichikawa et al. 2001; Pehek et al. 1993) and may normalize those presumed deficits in cortical dopamine function in schizophrenia remediated by nicotine administration via cigarette smoking (George et al. 2000a, 2002a).

Integrating Pharmacological and Behavioral Treatments for Smoking Cessation in Schizophrenia: Optimizing Treatment to Prevent the Onset of Smoking-Related Medical Illness

Despite the enhanced quality of life possibly afforded to individuals with schizophrenia with the use of atypical agents, it is becoming increasingly apparent that cigarette-smoking schizophrenic patients are vulnerable to developing smoking-related morbidity and mortality, including an increased risk of cardiovascular disease (Lichtermann et al. 2001; Tsuang et al. 1983) compared with the general population of smokers. Previous epidemiological studies have suggested that schizophrenic smokers are protected against the development of malignancies (Tsuang et al. 1980, 1983), and this was thought to relate to neuroleptic drug exposure (Mortensen 1987). In addition, there is evidence that urinary levels of the peptide bombesin, a possible marker of precancerous cigarette smoking–induced lung damage, are lower in schizophrenic patients compared with controls (Olincy et al. 1999). This reduction in urinary bombesin levels is independent of smoking status in schizophrenic patients, supporting the notion that schizophrenic patients may be less vulnerable to the development of cancer. However, several subsequent epidemiological studies have found no evidence for a decreased risk of lung cancer in schizophrenic patients or other patients with serious mental disorders (Lichtermann et al. 2001; Masterson and O'Shea 1984; Saku et al. 1995; Tsuang et al. 1983). In particular, the Finnish record linkage study noted the prevalence of lung cancer to be twice as high in patients with schizophrenia (Lichtermann et al. 2001). Previous studies may have been confounded by a selection bias in which rates of these medical illnesses in older schizophrenics were lower because most of this cohort had died from other causes related to their psychiatric illness (e.g., suicide) by the time they reached the age when cancer risk is substantially increased (50 years or older) (Allebeck 1989). Thus, disease prevention through smoking cessation or reduction in this population is an important public health issue, especially because schizophrenic patients constitute 1% of the population in the United States (Regier et al. 1990).

Although the interest of schizophrenic patients in smoking cessation is generally thought to be low, there are approximately 20%–40% whose desire to quit smoking is substantial (Addington et al. 1997, 1999; Ziedonis and George 1997), according to ratings of motivational level with the Stages of Change scale (e.g., preparation or action stages; Prochaska and DiClemente 1983). In many cases where smoking cessation is not possible, a reduction in smoking consumption (e.g., a "harm reduction" approach) might accrue some health benefits for schizophrenic smokers (Hughes 1998), but no studies have been published suggesting that reducing smoking can reduce the risk of developing smoking-related illness in nonpsychiatric or schizophrenic smokers. Thus, an understanding of biological and psychosocial factors that render schizophrenic patients at high risk for developing nicotine addiction and that contribute to their low intrinsic motivation to change smoking behaviors is critical to guiding efforts toward improving smoking cessation treatment in this population.

Experience in controlled treatment research studies for smoking cessation in schizophrenia has suggested the need to optimize both pharmacological and psychosocial interventions (George et al. 2000a, 2002b). Although atypical antipsychotic drugs may be one patient factor that predicts better smoking cessation or reduction outcomes, the reality is that schizophrenic patients need persistent efforts to encourage smoking cessation with the use of so-called motivational enhancement therapies and, once smoking abstinence has been achieved, require ongoing teaching in methods to prevent smoking relapse (Addington 1998; George et al. 2000a; Ziedonis and George 1997). In addition, it is helpful to educate patients about the dangers of smoking to their health, as they often know surprisingly little about the adverse effects of tobacco. Finally, drug refusal techniques are important because peer pressure is typically very high on these individuals to resume smoking after successful abstinence. In the experience of the Yale Program for Research in Smokers with Mental Illness, teaching assertiveness skills (in the context of social skills training) has been quite effective for those patients who can maintain high motivation to remain tobacco free.

Standard U.S. Food and Drug Administration–approved smoking cessation pharmacotherapies such as the NTP (Addington et al. 1998; George et al. 2000a) and sustained-release bupropion (Zyban) (Evins et al. 2001; George et al. 2002b; Weiner et al. 2001) appear to be safe and efficacious treatments for smoking cessation in schizophrenic patients during the course of controlled studies. Smoking cessation rates at the end of drug treatment with the NTP are in the range of 36%–42% (Addington et al. 1998; George et al. 2000a), and with bupropion, 11%–50% (Evins et al. 2001; George et al. 2002b; Weiner et al. 2001). These rates are modest compared with those achieved in nonschizophrenic control smokers (50%–75%) (Hughes et al. 1999) but may be improved when patients are prescribed atypical antipsychotic agents (George et al. 2000a, 2002b). Differences in study design, patient variables (e.g., level of motivation to quit smoking), medication dose (in the studies with bupropion, 150–300 mg/ day), and criteria used to determine smoking abstinence may explain the variability in cessation rates among these studies.

In studies that have used the NTP, patients are expected to stop all smoking when they begin use of the NTP, on the "quit date." Patients should be cautioned not to smoke while they are wearing the patch due to concerns about nicotine toxicity, symptoms of which can include tremor, nausea and vomiting, and dizziness, and in rare cases seizures, arrhythmias, and death. In our research clinic, we have not found nicotine toxicity to be a significant problem, but we tell patients if they must smoke, to remove the patch and wait 1–2 hours before resuming smoking. The craving to smoke and continuing withdrawal symptoms typically indicate incomplete nicotine replacement, and if necessary, another patch of 7–21 mg/ day can be added to therapy with the 21 mg/day NTP.

For Zyban, controlled studies have started dosing at 150 mg orally daily, increasing to 150 mg twice daily by the fourth day of treatment. The "quit date" is typically set once levels reach steady state, usually 3–4 days after beginning the full 300 mg/day dose. A history of seizures of any etiology is a contraindication to the use of Zyban, as indicated by the product labeling, and we recommend not exceeding the 300 mg/day dose, because some antipsychotic drugs may reduce seizure threshold. At the same time, Zyban at 150–300 mg/day does not appear to worsen positive symptoms of schizophrenia, and may reduce negative symptoms (Evins et al. 2001;

George et al. 2002b; Weiner et al. 2001). The typical duration of therapy studied in schizophrenic patients with these agents is 8–12 weeks; studies with longer durations of treatment in this population have not yet been conducted.

Conclusion

The following points about smoking in schizophrenic patients should be emphasized:

- The high rates of comorbid smoking in schizophrenic patients may relate to abnormal biology of nicotinic receptor systems and central dopamine pathways associated with this disorder. Hence, these patients may self-medicate clinical and cognitive deficits associated with schizophrenia that are nicotine responsive. These findings have profound implications for understanding the neurobiology of schizophrenic disorders, as well as for the development of better treatments for schizophrenia, and for addressing nicotine addiction in this disorder, given that these patients appear to be at increased risk for developing smoking-related medical illnesses.
- Motivation to quit smoking is often low in schizophrenic patients, and efforts need to be undertaken to increase awareness by both patients and their clinicians of the dangers of habitual tobacco smoking. Motivational enhancement and relapse prevention methods are the mainstays of behavioral treatment for nicotine addiction in these patients.
- There is increasing evidence from controlled studies that certain pharmacological agents do promote smoking reduction and cessation (e.g., atypical antipsychotic drugs, nicotine replacement, and bupropion), and that these agents can be used safely for the treatment of cigarette smoking and nicotine dependence in clinically stable patients with schizophrenic disorders. Although there is little evidence from controlled clinical studies that smoking cessation produces a deterioration of clinical function (e.g., positive and negative symptoms) in stabilized patients, clinicians should not attempt to get patients to quit smoking when they are clinically unstable because the likelihood of success is low.

References

Addington J: Group treatment for smoking cessation with schizophrenia. Psychiatr Serv 49:925–928, 1998

Addington J, el-Guebaly N, Addington D, et al: Readiness to stop smoking in schizophrenia. Can J Psychol 42:49–52, 1997

Addington J, el-Guebaly N, Campbell W, et al: Smoking cessation treatment for patients with schizophrenia. Am J Psychiatry 155:974–976, 1998

Addington J, el-Guebaly N, Duchak V, et al: Using measures of readiness to change in individuals with schizophrenia. Am J Drug Alcohol Abuse 25:151–161, 1999

Adler LE, Hoffer LD, Wiser A, et al: Normalization of auditory physiology by cigarette smoking in schizophrenic patients. Am J Psychiatry 150:1856–1861, 1993

Adler LE, Hoffer LD, Waldo M, et al: Schizophrenia, sensory gating and nicotinic receptors. Schizophr Bull 24:189–202, 1998

Allebeck P: Schizophrenia: a life-shortening disease. Schizophr Bull 15:81–89, 1989

American Psychiatric Association: Diagnostic and Statistical Manual of Mental Disorders, 4th Edition, Text Revision. Washington, DC, American Psychiatric Association, 2000

Arnsten AF: Through the looking glass: differential noradrenergic modulation of prefrontal cortical function. Neural Plast 7:133–146, 2000

Balfour DJK, Fagerstrom KO: Pharmacology of nicotine and its therapeutic use in smoking cessation and neurodegenerative disorders. Pharmacol Ther 72:51–81, 1996

Chong SA, Choo HL: Smoking among Chinese patients with schizophrenia. Aust N Z J Psychiatry 30:350–353, 1996

Collins AC, Luo Y, Selvang S, et al: Sensitivity to nicotine and brain nicotinic receptors are altered by chronic nicotine and mecamylamine infusion. J Pharmacol Exp Ther 271:125–133, 1994

Dalack GW, Meador-Woodruff JH: Smoking, smoking withdrawal and schizophrenia: case reports and a review of the literature. Schizophr Res 22:133–141, 1996

Dalack GW, Meador-Woodruff JH: Acute feasibility and safety of a smoking reduction strategy for smokers with schizophrenia. Nicotine Tob Res 1:53–57, 1999

Dalack GW, Healy DJ, Meador-Woodruff JH: Nicotine dependence and schizophrenia: clinical phenomenon and laboratory findings. Am J Psychiatry 155:1490–1501, 1998

Dalack GW, Becks L, Hill E, et al: Nicotine withdrawal and psychiatric symptoms in cigarette smokers with schizophrenia. Neuropsychopharmacology 21:195–202, 1999

de Leon J, Dadvand M, Canuso C, et al: Schizophrenia and smoking: an epidemiological survey in a state hospital. Am J Psychiatry 152:453–455, 1995

Decina P, Caracci G, Sandik R, et al: Cigarette smoking and neuroleptic-induced parkinsonism. Biol Psychiatry 28:502–508, 1990

Diwan A, Castine M, Pomerleau CS, et al: Differential prevalence of cigarette smoking in patients with schizophrenia vs. mood disorders. Schizophr Res 33:113–118, 1998 el-Guebaly N, Hodgins D: Schizophrenia and substance abuse: prevalence issues. Can J Psychiatry 37:704–710, 1992

Evins AE, Mays VK, Rigotti NA, et al: A pilot trial of bupropion added to cognitive behavioral therapy for smoking cessation in schizophrenia. Nicotine Tob Res 3:397–403, 2001

Fowler JS, Volkow ND, Wang G-J, et al: Inhibition of monoamine oxidase B in the brains of smokers. Nature 379:733–736, 1996a

Fowler JS, Volkow ND, Wang G-J, et al: Brain monoamine oxidase A: inhibition by cigarette smoke. Proc Natl Acad Sci U S A 93:14065–14069, 1996b

Freedman R, Coon H, Myles-Worsley M, et al: Linkage of a neurophysiological deficit in schizophrenia to a chromosome 15 locus. Proc Natl Acad Sci U S A 94:587–592, 1997

George TP, Vessicchio JC: Nicotine addiction and schizophrenia. Psychiatric Times 18:39–42, 2001

George TP, Sernyak MJ, Ziedonis DM, et al: Effects of clozapine on smoking in chronic schizophrenic outpatients. J Clin Psychiatry 56:344–346, 1995

George TP, Verrico CD, Roth RH: Effects of repeated nicotine pre-treatment on mesoprefontal dopaminergic and behavioral responses to acute footshock stress. Brain Res 801:36–49, 1998

George TP, Zeidonis DM, Feingold A, et al: Nicotine transdermal patch and atypical antipsychotic medications for smoking cessation in schizophrenia. Am J Psychiatry 157:1835–1842, 2000a

George TP, Verrico CD, Xu L, et al: Effects of repeated nicotine administration and footshock stress on rat mesoprefrontal dopamine systems: evidence for opioid mechanisms. Neuropsychopharmacology 23:79–88, 2000b

George TP, Verrico CD, Picciotto MR, et al: Nicotinic modulation of mesoprefrontal dopamine systems: pharmacologic and neuroanatomic characterization. J Pharmacol Exp Ther 295:58–66, 2000c

George TP, Vessicchio JC, Termine A, et al: A laboratory study of nicotinic receptor mechanisms and cognitive function in schizophrenia. Paper presented at the 40th annual meeting of the American College of Neuropsychopharmacology, Waikoloa, HI, 2001

George TP, Vessicchio JC, Termine A, et al: Effects of smoking abstinence on visuospatial working memory function in schizophrenia. Neuropsychopharmacology 26:75–85, 2002a

George TP, Vessicchio JC, Termine A, et al: A placebo-controlled study of bupropion for smoking cessation in schizophrenia. Biol Psychiatry 52:53–61, 2002b

Goff DC, Henderson DC, Amico E: Cigarette smoking in schizophrenia: relationship to psychopathology and medication side effects. Am J Psychiatry 149:1189–1194, 1992

Hall RG, Duhamel M, McClanahan R, et al: Level of functioning, severity of illness, and smoking status among chronic psychiatric patients. J Nerv Ment Dis 183:468–471, 1995

Hamera E, Schneider JK, Deviney S: Alcohol, cannabis, nicotine and caffeine use and symptom distress in schizophrenia. J Nerv Ment Dis 183:559–565, 1995

Hughes JR: Harm-reduction approaches to smoking: the need for data. Am J Prev Med 15:9–16, 1998

Hughes JR, Hatsukami DK, Mitchell JE, et al: Prevalence of smoking among psychiatric outpatients. Am J Psychiatry 143:993–997, 1986

Hughes JR, Goldstein MG, Hurt RD, et al: Recent advances in the pharmacotherapy of smoking. JAMA 281:72–76, 1999

Ichikawa J, Ishii H, Bonaccorso S, et al: 5-HT(2A) and D(2) receptor blockade increases cortical DA release via 5-HT(1A) receptor activation: a possible mechanism of atypical antipsychotic-induced cortical dopamine release. J Neurochem 76:1521–1531, 2001

Kelly C, McCredie RG: Smoking habits, current symptoms, and premorbid characteristics of schizophrenic patients in Nithsdale, Scotland. Am J Psychiatry 156:1751–1757, 1999

Knable MB, Weinberger DR: Dopamine, the prefrontal cortex and schizophrenia. J Psychopharmacol 11:123–131, 1997

Kumari V, Checkly SA, Gray JA: Effects of cigarette smoking on prepulse inhibition of the acoustic startle reflex in healthy male smokers. Psychopharmacology (Berl) 128:54–60, 1996

Kumari V, Soni W, Sharma T: Normalization of information processing deficits in schizophrenia with clozapine. Am J Psychiatry 156:1046–1051, 1999

Lasser K, Boyd JW, Woolhander S, et al: Smoking and mental illness: a population-based prevalence study. JAMA 284:2606–2610, 2000

Levin ED, Wilson W, Rose J, et al: Nicotine-haloperidol interactions and cognitive performance in schizophrenics. Neuropsychopharmacology 15:429–436, 1996

Lichtermann D, Ekelund E, Pukkala E, et al: Incidence of cancer among persons with schizophrenia and their relatives. Arch Gen Psychiatry 58:573–578, 2001

Light GA, Geyer MA, Clementz BA, et al: Normal P50 supression in schizophrenia patients treated with atypical antipsychotic drugs. Am J Psychiatry 157:767–771, 2000

Masterson E, O'Shea B: Smoking and malignancy in schizophrenia. Br J Psychiatry 145:429–432, 1984

McEvoy JP, Brown S: Smoking in first-episode patients with schizophrenia. Am J Psychiatry 156:1120–1121, 1999

McEvoy J, Freudenreich O, McGee M, et al: Clozapine decreases smoking in patients with chronic schizophrenia. Biol Psychiatry 37:550–552, 1995a

McEvoy J, Freudenreich O, Levin E, et al: Haloperidol increases smoking in patients with schizophrenia. Psychopharmacology (Berl) 119:124–126, 1995b

McEvoy JP, Freudenreich O, Wilson WH: Smoking and therapeutic response to clozapine in patients with schizophrenia. Biol Psychiatry 46:125–129, 1999

McGehee DS, Heath MJ, Gelber S, et al: Nicotinic enhancment of fast excitatory synaptic transmission in CNS by presynaptic receptors. Science 269:1692–1696, 1995

Menza MA, Grossman M, Van Horn M, et al: Smoking and movement disorders in psychiatric patients. Biol Psychiatry 30:109–115, 1991

Meyer JM: Individual changes in clozapine levels after smoking. cessation: results and a predictive model. J Clin Psychopharmacol 21:569–574, 2001

Mortensen PB: Neuroleptic medication and other factors modifying cancer risk in schizophrenic patients. Acta Psychiatr Scand 75:585–590, 1987

Nagamoto HT, Adler LE, Waldo MC, et al: Gating of auditory P50 in schizophrenics: unique effects of clozapine. Biol Psychiatry 40:181–188, 1996

O'Farrell TJ, Connors GJ, Upper D: Addictive behaviors among hospitalized psychiatric patients. Addict Behav 8:329–333, 1983

Olincy A, Leonard S, Young DA, et al: Decreased bombesin peptide response to cigarette smoking in schizophrenia. Neuropsychopharmacology 20:52–59, 1999

Park S, Knopnick C, McGurk S, et al: Nicotine impairs spatial working memory while leaving spatial attention intact. Neuropsychopharmacology 22:200–209, 2000

Parwani A, Duncan EJ, Bartlett E, et al: Impaired prepulse inhibition of acoustic startle in schizophrenia. Biol Psychiatry 47:662–669, 2000

Pehek EA, Meltzer HY, Yamamoto BK: The atypical antipsychotic drug amperozide enhances cortical and striatal dopamine efflux. Eur J Pharmacol 240:107–109, 1993

Perry PJ, Miller DD, Arndt SV, et al: Haloperidol dosing requirements: the contributions of smoking and nonlinear pharmacokinetics. J Clin Psychopharmacol 13:46–51, 1993

Perry PJ, Bever KA, Arndt S, et al: Relationship between patient variables and plasma clozapine concentrations: a dosing nomogram. Biol Psychiatry 44:733–738, 1998

Picciotto MR, Caldarone BJ, King SL, et al: Nicotinic receptors in the brain: links between molecular biology and behavior. Neuropsychopharmacology 22:451–465, 2000

Prochaska JO, DiClemente CC: Stages and processes of self-change of smoking: toward an integrative model of change. J Consult Clin Psychol 51:390–395, 1983

Regier DA, Farmer ME, Rae DS, et al: Comorbidity of mental disorders with alcohol and other drug abuse: results from the Epidemiologic Catchment Area (ECA) study. JAMA 264:2511–2518, 1990

Saku M, Tokudome S, Ikeda M, et al: Mortality in psychiatric patients, with a specific focus on cancer mortality associated with schizophrenia. Int J Epidemiol 24:366–372, 1995

Sandyk R: Cigarette smoking: effects on cognitive functions and drug-induced parkinsonism in chronic schizophrenia. Int J Neurosci 70:193–197, 1993

Seppala NH, Leinonen EV, Lehtonen ML, et al: Clozapine serum concentrations are lower in smoking than in non-smoking schizophrenic patients. Pharmacol Toxicol 85:244–246, 1999

Swerdlow NR, Caine SB, Braff DL, et al: The neural substrates of sensorimotor gating of the startle reflex: a review of recent findings and their implications. J Psychopharmacol 6:176–190, 1992

Tsuang MT, Woolson RF, Fleming JA: Premature deaths in schizophrenia and affective disorders: an analysis of survival curves and variables affecting the shortened survival. Arch Gen Psychiatry 37:979–983, 1980

Tsuang MT, Perkins K, Simpson JC: Physical diseases in schizophrenia and affective disorder. J Clin Psychiatry 44:42–46, 1983

Vocci F, DeWit H (eds): NIDA/CPDD Consensus Statement on Evaluation of Outcomes for Pharmacotherapy of Substance Abuse/Dependence. Rockville, MD, National Institute on Drug Abuse, 1999

Weiner E, Ball MP, Summerfelt A, et al: Effects of sustained-release bupropion and supportive group therapy on cigarette consumption in patients with schizophrenia. Am J Psychiatry 158:635–637, 2001

Williams GV, Goldman-Rakic PS: Modulation of memory fields by dopamine D_1 receptors in the prefrontal cortex. Nature 376:572–575, 1995

Yassa R, Lal S, Korpassy A, Ally J: Nicotine exposure and tardive dyskinesia. Biol Psychiatry 30:109–115, 1987

Zahrt J, Taylor JR, Matthew RG, et al: Supranormal stimulation of D_1 receptors in the rodent prefrontal cortex impairs spatial working memory performance. J Neurosci 17:8528–8535, 1997

Ziedonis DM, Kosten TR, Glazer WM, et al: Nicotine dependence and schizophrenia. Hosp Community Psychiatry 45:204–206, 1994

Ziedonis DM, George TP: Schizophrenia and nicotine use: report of a pilot smoking cessation program and review of neurobiological and clinical issues. Schizophr Bull 23:247–254, 1997

Chapter 6

Glucose Intolerance and Diabetes in Schizophrenia

David C. Henderson, M.D.

Elissa Powers Ettinger, M.D.

Introduction

In recent years, tremendous progress has been made in the treatment of schizophrenia and other psychotic disorders. In particular, the introduction of atypical antipsychotic agents has helped numerous patients gain control of both the positive and negative symptoms of schizophrenia. Recent studies also suggest that the newer antipsychotic agents increase compliance, prevent relapse (Csernansky et al. 2002), and may offer improvement in the treatment of cognitive dysfunction (Meltzer 2001). These treatment successes, combined with a lower risk of extrapyramidal symptoms (e.g., parkinsonism), have led many psychiatrists to favor the newer, atypical antipsychotic medications over the older, typical agents.

The use of atypical antipsychotic medications, however, has not proven trouble free. More specifically, there have been numerous reports in the psychiatric and medical literature suggesting an association between atypical antipsychotic agents and impaired glucose metabolism (Henderson 2001b; Mir and Taylor 2001). After a brief review of the pathophysiology of diabetes mellitus, especially type II diabetes mellitus, and its short- and long-term medical consequences, this chapter examines the prevalence of glucose intolerance and diabetes in individuals with schizophrenia compared with the general population before and following the introduction of typical and atypical antipsychotic medications. Finally, recommendations for monitoring and screening for glucose intolerance and diabetes in schizophrenia patients will be made.

Glucose Intolerance and Diabetes Mellitus

Diagnostic Criteria and the Pathophysiology of Diabetes Mellitus

Before a discussion of the relationship between schizophrenia and diabetes, it is helpful to define diabetes and glucose intolerance, both of which are characterized by problems in glucose-insulin regulation. According to the American Diabetes Association (ADA), if an individual has the typical symptoms of diabetes, such as polyuria, polydipsia, and unexplained weight loss, plus a casual plasma glucose level ≥200 mg/dL (11.1 mmol/L), a fasting plasma glucose level ≥126 mg/dL (7.0 mmol/L), or a 2-hour plasma glucose level ≥200 mg/dL (11.1 mmol/L) post 75 g oral glucose load, then he or she has diabetes mellitus (Expert Committee on the Diagnosis and Classification of Diabetes Mellitus 2000). Similarly, if an individual has a 2-hour plasma glucose level ≥140 mg/dL and <200 mg/dL post 75 g oral glucose load, he or she is said to have impaired glucose tolerance (Expert Committee on the Diagnosis and Classification of Diabetes Mellitus 2000). Impaired fasting glucose is defined as a level from 110 to 125 mg/dL; fasting glucose values under 110 mg/dL are considered to be in the normal range.

Two pathophysiological processes can lead to the development of glucose intolerance and diabetes mellitus: 1) a problem with insulin secretion, as in type I and the later stages of type II diabetes mellitus, and 2) a problem with insulin action, otherwise known as insulin resistance, as seen in type II diabetes mellitus (Lebovitz 2001). In the first case, the beta cells of the pancreas have been destroyed by an autoimmune process, and hyperglycemia occurs because not enough insulin is secreted to facilitate glucose uptake in skeletal muscle tissue, inhibit glucose production in hepatic tissue, and suppress lipolysis in adipose tissue. In type II diabetes mellitus, although there may be enough insulin secreted, insulin resistance prevents the insulin from working at the sites of skeletal muscle, hepatic, and adipose tissues. Indeed, there may even be a reactive hyperinsulinemia, which may help control plasma glucose levels initially, but eventually the beta cells in the pancreas begin to deteriorate at a genetically determined rate, and the compensatory hyperinsulinemia decreases (Lebovitz 2001). As this occurs, the postprandial plasma glucose levels increase progressively, and the individual progresses from normal glucose tolerance to impaired glucose tolerance to type II diabetes mellitus. Thus, patients with type II diabetes mellitus have both insulin resistance and an insulin secretory deficit due to decreased beta cell function.

Both type I and type II diabetes mellitus are diseases with mutifactorial inheritance. Researchers are confident that no single gene causes type I or type II diabetes, and that development of this heterogeneous group of disorders is likely the result of multiple genetic and environmental factors. For example, the interaction of genetic factors such as beta cell abnormalities and a predisposition for central obesity with excess caloric intake, high fat ingestion, and decreased physical activity can lead to type II diabetes in some individuals (Lebovitz 2001).

Drugs are another environmental factor that can cause diabetes mellitus either by destroying the beta cells in the pancreas or by causing insulin resistance by one of the following mechanisms: 1) increasing appetite and caloric intake, leading to obesity; 2) altering fat distribution (central obesity is a risk factor for diabetes mellitus); 3) decreasing physical activity because of increased sedation; 4) decreasing oxidative metabolism in tissues; 5) interfering with the insulin action cascade; 6) increasing counterregulatory hormones; or 7) increasing free fatty acid release from adipose tissue (Lebovitz 2001). Later in this chapter, we discuss the possible mechanisms by which atypical antipsychotic medications may cause glucose intolerance or diabetes mellitus, exacerbate existing diabetes, or induce diabetic ketoacidosis in patients with schizophrenia.

Medical Complications of Glucose Intolerance and Diabetes Mellitus

Hyperglycemia and diabetes mellitus are associated with acute and chronic complications associated with significant morbidity and mortality. Diabetic ketoacidosis (DKA), an acute complication of diabetes mellitus, is seen more often in patients with type I than in patients with type II diabetes mellitus and is a serious and potentially fatal complication. Ketoacidosis is defined by low serum pH (≤ 7.35), low serum bicarbonate levels (≤ 15), and an anion gap in the presence of ketonemia (Westphal 1996). The diabetic patient is also susceptible to a variety of chronic complications that affect the cardiovascular system, nervous system, eyes, kidneys, and wound-healing capabilities.

Most of these complications are a result of microvascular and macrovascular disease that is more extensive and appears much earlier in the diabetic patient than in the general population (Newcomer 2001).

Macrovascular disease in the form of atherosclerosis increases the risk of cardiovascular and cerebrovascular events such as myocardial infarction and stroke, accounting for much of the disability and death among diabetic patients (Haupt and Newcomer 2001; Henderson 2001a). According to data amassed by Gerstein and his colleagues from large samples of patients without diabetes (Gerstein et al. 1999), even modest increases in fasting plasma glucose levels that do not meet the diagnostic criteria for diabetes mellitus put patients at increased risk for coronary artery disease, myocardial infarction, and other vascular problems. In peripheral sites, atherosclerosis can cause claudication and "diabetic foot," a condition in which patients develop nonhealing ulcers that are prone to infection on their lower extremities and feet as a result of vascular insufficiency and sensory deficits from impairments in the peripheral nervous system. Diabetic neuropathy is a complication that contributes significantly to morbidity in diabetic patients, because it not only contributes to diabetic foot but can affect any part of the nervous system, resulting in sensory deficits, paresthesias, motor abnormalities, or autonomic dysfunction (Henderson 2001a). A large percentage of diabetic patients also experience ophthalmic complications such as diabetic retinopathy and diseases of the anterior chamber that affect vision (e.g., cataracts), leading to blindness and significant disability in diabetic patients.

Finally, many diabetic patients suffer a great deal from microvascular- and macrovascular-induced nephropathy, which can cause hypertension, proteinuria, and a decrease in the glomerular filtration rate, leading to renal failure. Indeed, diabetic nephropathy accounts for approximately 25% of end-stage renal failure cases in the United States (Expert Committee on the Diagnosis and Classification of Diabetes Mellitus 2000) and is a leading cause of morbidity and mortality in diabetic patients.

In summary, it is clear that diabetes is a disease associated with considerable medical morbidity and mortality.

Diabetes and Glucose Intolerance in Schizophrenic Patients in the Pre-antipsychotic Era

Early reports dating back to the 1920s, before the use of antipsychotic agents, suggest that individuals with schizophrenia and other psychotic disorders exhibited an elevated risk for developing glucose intolerance or diabetes mellitus (Braceland et al. 1945; Brambilla et al. 1976; Haupt and Newcomer 2001; Marinow 1971; Schwartz and Munoz 1968; Waitzkin 1966a, 1966b). Specifically, the reports indicate a pattern of insulin resistance in schizophrenic patients independent of adverse medication effects (Haupt and Newcomer 2001). These studies, however, suffer from several methodological problems: there are flaws in the diagnostic criteria for schizophrenia, and they do not control for age, weight, fat distribution, ethnicity, diet, or exercise, all of which are variables now known to play a role in an individual's risk for developing glucoregulatory disturbances (Haupt and Newcomer 2001). Because no well-controlled studies exist, whether individuals with schizophrenia, when unmedicated, are at increased risk for developing diabetes compared with the general population remains a matter of debate.

Conventional Antipsychotic Agents, Diabetes, and Glucose Intolerance

Conventional antipsychotic agents, which have primarily antidopaminergic activity, may alter glucose–insulin homeostasis (Hagg et al. 1998). In particular, the low-potency phenothiazines may induce diabetes mellitus or aggravate existing diabetes mellitus (Hagg et al. 1998; Haupt and Newcomer 2001). Because of this finding, chlorpromazine has been used to prevent hypoglycemia in patients with malignant insulinoma. Furthermore, chlorpromazine has been shown to induce hyperglycemia in healthy volunteers as well as in patients with latent diabetes (Hagg et al. 1998).

Other conventional antipsychotic agents, such as the higher-potency agent haloperidol, are associated with a decrease in the prevalence rate of diabetes in the schizophrenia population. For example, Mukherjee et al. (1996) found an overall diabetes prevalence rate of 15% in 95 patients with schizophrenia. In patients younger than 50 years, there were no cases of diabetes mellitus. For patients ages 50 to 59 years, however, the prevalence rate was 12.9%, and for patients ages 60 to 69 years the prevalence rate was 18.9%. Finally, for those ages 70 to 74 years the prevalence rate was 16.7%. Controlling for age, gender, and cumulative duration of anti-psychotic treatment, medication-free patients were more likely to develop diabetes mellitus than those receiving treatment with conventional agents (Mukherjee et al. 1996). Notably, the prevalence rates quoted in Mukherjee's study exceeded those expected for type II diabetes mellitus in the general population, lending further evidence to the argument that schizophrenia may indeed be an independent risk factor for the development of diabetes mellitus (Henderson 2001b).

In summary, examination of reports discussing the prevalence rates of diabetes mellitus or impaired glucose tolerance in schizophrenic patients shows that among the conventional antipsychotic agents, the effects of glucose regulation may vary in magnitude across individual agents. Specifically, the phenothiazines may increase a patient's susceptibility to developing diabetes mellitus, but there is no significant association between diabetes mellitus and the use of other conventional antipsychotic medications.

Diabetes and Glucose Intolerance in Patients With Schizophrenia Taking Atypical Antipsychotic Medications

The greatest benefit of the introduction of the atypical antipsychotic medications as a group—clozapine, olanzapine, quetiapine, risperidone, and ziprasidone—has been the improvement in the treatment of negative symptoms and concomitant improvements in cognitive function (Meltzer 2001). This improvement in cognitive function, which includes the aspects of executive function, verbal fluency, attention, and memory and learning, can lead to improved functioning in both home and work environments (Meltzer 2001). Furthermore, the atypical antipsychotic agents have been shown to decrease depression, and clozapine in particular has been shown to decrease suicidality in schizophrenic patients (Meltzer 2001). Clozapine has also proven to be the most effective drug for the treatment of patients with refractory schizophrenia. A 6-week trial produced a response rate of 30% of patients with treatment-resistant disease (Kane et al. 1988), which increased to 60% after 6 months of therapy (Meltzer et al. 1990).

However, improvements in efficacy for symptoms of schizophrenia have not come without cost. Many atypical antipsychotic agents are associated with significant weight gain, particularly the development of central obesity, which has an adverse effect on health and medication compliance (Meyer 2001). Allison et al. (1999) performed a meta-analysis and estimated that the average weight change for subjects treated with antipsychotic agents over a 10-week period was 0.74 kg reduction with placebo, 0.39 kg reduction with molindone, 3.19 kg increase with thioridazine, 4.45 kg increase with clozapine, 4.15 kg increase with olanzapine, 2.92 kg increase with sertindole, 2.10 kg increase with risperidone, and 0.04 kg increase with ziprasidone. Significant weight gain during atypical antipsychotic therapy can contribute to comorbid conditions such as coronary artery disease, hypertension, and type II diabetes mellitus (Meyer 2001).

There have been numerous reports in the medical and psychiatric literature of cases linking the use of atypical antipsychotic agents to the development of glucose intolerance, new-onset diabetes mellitus, DKA, and exacerbation of existing type I or type II diabetes mellitus, even in patients who are not obese (Henderson 2001a; Mir and Taylor 2001). Koller and colleagues from the U.S. Food and Drug Administration (FDA) Research program conducted a Medwatch surveillance program analysis and reported 384 reports of clozapine-related diabetes (Koller et al. 2001), of which 242 were new-onset diabetes reports and 54 were reports of exacerbation in patients with preexisting diabetes. The report also identified 80 cases of clozapine-induced probable DKA and 25 deaths. Of note, the majority of DKA episodes occurred within the first 6 months of clozapine treatment, and one patient developed diabetes mellitus immediately after he accidentally took a 500 mg dose of clozapine. Koller also published data on olanzapine and found a total of 289 cases, of which 225 were new-onset diabetes mellitus, with 100 cases of DKA and 25 deaths (Koller and Doraiswamy 2002). Given that the Medwatch surveillance program is able to identify only a small percentage of cases, it is likely that the prevalence of clozapine- and olanzapine-induced diabetes mellitus and DKA is much greater, and there appears to be serious potential risk associated with the use of these agents for the development of diabetes mellitus and DKA.

Among the published literature on this issue, Popli et al. (1997) described four cases in which schizophrenic patients being treated with clozapine had exacerbation of their existing diabetes mellitus or de novo diabetes mellitus not attributable to weight gain. Wirshing et al. (1998) described four cases of clozapine-associated diabetes and two cases of olanzapine-associated diabetes, with weight gain during atypical therapy noted in only 50% of these cases. Hagg et al. (1998), using an oral glucose tolerance test (OGTT), found that 12% of patients treated with clozapine developed type II diabetes and 10% developed impaired glucose tolerance, compared with 6% and 3%, respectively, of patients treated with conventional depot antipsychotic medications. Another group investigating the association between the atypical antipsychotic agents and diabetes mellitus, led by Melkersson, found elevated fasting insulin levels and reduced growth hormone–dependent insulin-like growth factor I when they compared 28 patients with schizophrenia on therapy with conventional antipsychotic agents and 13 patients treated with clozapine, suggesting insulin resistance with secondary increased hyperinsulinemia related to clozapine therapy (Melkersson et al. 1999).

Finally, a group at Harvard conducted a 5-year naturalistic study examining, in 101 patients with schizophrenia treated with clozapine, the incidence of treatment-emergent diabetes in relation to other factors such as body weight gain, lipid level abnormalities, age, clozapine dose, and concomitant treatment with valproic acid (Henderson et al. 2000a). Patients with diabetes prior to clozapine initiation required nearly a twofold increase in insulin requirement or a switch to insulin from an oral hypoglycemic agent after begining clozapine. In the study, the mean age at the time of clozapine initiation was 36.4 years; 26.8% of the patients were women, and 91% were Caucasian. The mean baseline weight was 175.5 pounds, and the mean body mass index was 26.9 kg/m^2. During the 5-year follow-up, 30 patients (36%) were diagnosed with diabetes. Patients experienced significant weight gain that continued until approximately month 46 from the beginning of clozapine treatment, but weight gain was not a significant risk factor for the development of diabetes in this study.

Clozapine is not the only atypical antipsychotic agent that has been associated with the development of glucose intolerance, diabetes mellitus, or DKA or exacerbation of existing diabetes mellitus. As noted previously, Wirshing et al. (1998) reported two cases of olanzapine-associated diabetes. Subsequently, Goldstein et al. (1999) described several cases of olanzapine-induced new-onset diabetes mellitus and DKA, of which the majority occurred within the first 3 months of treatment with olanzapine. It is important to note, however, that among the cases reported by Goldstein et al., some were complicated by concomitant treatment with valproic acid, which is believed to contribute to polycystic ovary disease and centripetal obesity, both of which can also lead to diabetes mellitus (Isojarvi et al. 1993, 1998).

Lindenmayer and Patel reported another olanzapine-induced case of new-onset diabetes, in which the patient developed diabetes mellitus 8 months after initiation of olanzapine treatment (Lindenmayer and Patel 1999). The same patient had complete resolution of her diabetes after the drug was discontinued (Lindenmayer and Patel 1999). Fertig et al. (1998) reported a case in which an obese African American man developed new-onset diabetes mellitus after only 6 weeks of treatment with olanzapine. His diabetes also resolved after discontinuation of the drug, and it returned within 8 days after olanzapine treatment was reinitiated.

Olanzapine therapy has also been associated with the development of DKA, as noted in a report by Gatta et al. (1999). In that case, olanzapine-associated diabetic ketoacidosis required the discontinuation of olanzapine and necessitated the use of insulin. The patient's diabetes completely resolved within 15 days of discontinuation of the olanzapine.

There have also been a few reports linking the atypical antipsychotic agents risperidone and quetiapine to new-onset diabetes mellitus and glucose intolerance, but not nearly as many as those described for clozapine and olanzapine (Henderson 2001b). Griffiths and Springuel (2001), using the Canadian Adverse Drug Reaction Monitoring Program, reported 37 cases of glucose metabolism disorders suspected to be associated with atypical antipsychotic agents. With clozapine there were 8 cases of diabetes mellitus, 5 cases of DKA, and 4 cases of hyperglycemia. For olanzapine 2 cases of diabetes mellitus were reported, along with 3 cases of DKA, 2 cases of diabetic coma, and 3 cases of hyperglycemia. For quetiapine, 1 case of diabetes mellitus and 2 cases of DKA were reported. Finally, for risperidone, 1 case of diabetes mellitus, 1 case of labile blood glucose levels, 3 cases of hyperglycemia, and 2 cases of hypoglycemia in patients with a previous history of diabetes mellitus were reported. Of note, there were 3 deaths from the 10 cases of DKA.

Recently, Wirshing et al. (2001) reported two cases of new-onset diabetes in risperidone-treated patients. Both subjects were African American, were overweight or obese prior to risperidone initiation, and gained significant weight while receiving treatment with the risperidone. These cases highlight the importance of understanding risk factors for diabetes in patients receiving treatment with atypical antipsychotic agents.

Finally, Fryburg et al. (2000) reported a double-blind controlled trial comparing olanzapine and ziprasidone therapy on the basis of metabolic indices. On a comparison of baseline to 6-week follow-up, olanzapine subjects showed a significant increase in body weight, fasting serum insulin, cholesterol, triglycerides, and a parameter for insulin resistance, suggesting a worsening insulin resistance in the olanzapine group but not the ziprasidone group.

All of the reports indicate that the strength of the association between the atypical antipsychotic medications and disturbances in glucose regulation can vary across the different medications, with many more cases of medication-induced hyperglycemia, diabetes mellitus, or DKA occurring with clozapine and olanzapine treatment than with treatment with the atypical agents risperidone, quetiapine, and ziprasidone (Haupt and Newcomer 2001). Also, it is important to recognize that the reports of DKA associated with clozapine and olanzapine treatments and the increased incidence of de novo type II diabetes mellitus may represent two distinct populations with varying risks for developing the diseases (Henderson 2001a).

Mechanisms by Which the Atypical Antipsychotic Agents May Cause Diabetes Mellitus

There are a number of ways in which the atypical antipsychotic medications could lead to hyperglycemia and diabetes mellitus. As discussed earlier in this chapter, decreased sensitivity (increased resistance) to insulin and decreased insulin secretion as a result of decreased beta cell function are involved in the development of type II diabetes mellitus. A few controlled studies suggest that the atypical antipsychotic medications affect insulin resistance rather than causing a primary defect in insulin secretion (Henderson et al. 2000b; Selke et al. 2000). The insulin resistance seen during atypical antipsychotic treatment may be a result of increased central adiposity, or it may arise from the direct effect of the medication's action on the glucose transporter function (Haupt and Newcomer 2001). Dwyer et al. (1999) studied the effects of atypical antipsychotic agents on glucose transporter function. They suggested that a structure–function relationship exists in which similar drugs, such as clozapine and olanzapine, achieve relatively higher intracellular concentrations and bind to, and thus interfere with, the function of the glucose transporter proteins (Haupt and Newcomer 2001).

Another mechanism by which the atypical antipsychotic agents may lead to hyperglycemia and diabetes mellitus is antagonism of the serotonin 5-HT_{1A} receptors. Antagonism of the 5-HT_{1A} receptors may decrease pancreatic beta cell responsiveness to blood sugar levels, resulting in disturbances in glucose metabolism secondary to decreased insulin secretion (Wirshing et al. 1998). Melkersson and colleagues, however, found that patients treated with olanzapine had higher fasting insulin levels on comparison of baseline to 5-month follow-up, suggesting that impaired beta cell function is an unlikely cause for olanzapine-associated diabetes mellitus (Melkersson et al. 2000). Their group found that although 11 of 14 olanzapine-treated patients (79%) were normoglycemic, and only 3 showed increased blood glucose values, the majority of patients (10 of 14, or 71%) had insulin levels above the normal limit. The report also noted increased rates of hyperleptinemia, hypertriglyceridemia, and hypercholesterolemia. In short, Melkersson and colleagues found that olanzapine treatment was associated with weight gain and elevated levels of insulin, leptin, and blood glucose levels as well as insulin resistance, with 3 patients diagnosed with diabetes mellitus (Melkersson et al. 2000). The elevated insulin values argue against the theory that antagonism of the serotonin receptors by some atypical anti-psychotic agents, a property that could theoretically lead to decreased beta cell insulin production, causes hyperglycemia and diabetes mellitus. It is also worth noting that olanzapine has little affinity for 5-HT_{1A} receptors.

Central obesity is a significant risk factor for the development of type II diabetes mellitus in schizophrenic patients as well as in the general population. The risk for the development of type II diabetes in mildly obese individuals has been reported as 2-fold, in moderately obese individuals

5-fold, and in severely obese individuals 10-fold (Pi-Snyder 1993). It seems, however, that the duration of obesity is a greater determinant of risk than simply being obese. That is, if a patient gains a considerable amount of weight and maintains this weight, his or her risk of developing hyperglycemia or type II diabetes mellitus appears to be increased (Henderson 2001a).

Notably, in several of the case studies and research studies mentioned in this chapter, weight gain was not associated with the development of diabetes mellitus or DKA during atypical antipsychotic therapy. Indeed, many of the individuals who developed diabetes mellitus or DKA were of normal weight. Thus, while all obese individuals are at increased risk for the development of type II diabetes mellitus, the added obesity caused by the atypical antipsychotic medications does not appear to be the sole reason for the development of diabetes mellitus or DKA in schizophrenia patients. Nevertheless, if a schizophrenia patient gains a considerable amount of weight and maintains that weight, his or her risk of developing type II diabetes is significantly increased.

Monitoring and Screening Recommendations

The development of glucose intolerance and diabetes mellitus may be a very serious comorbid complication of treatment with antipsychotic agents, thus contributing to the morbidity and mortality in schizophrenia patients. The development of hyperglycemia in schizophrenia patients often goes unrecognized, as it does in approximately 50% of the general population who have this condition. Because patients taking antipsychotic medications may be at increased risk for developing diabetes, close monitoring and screening for obesity and hyperglycemia are imperative for individualizing treatment decisions and reducing the risks of morbidity and mortality (Haupt and Newcomer 2001). Before starting treatment with an atypical antipsychotic, the clinician should perform a risk factor assessment for diabetes mellitus and other metabolic disorders. This risk assessment should include baseline serum lipid and glucose values (preferably fasting), weight, body mass index, age, ethnicity, family history of diabetes in a first-degree relative, level of physical activity, and diet (Expert Committee on the Diagnosis and Classification of Diabetes Mellitus 2000).

The American Diabetes Association (2000) recommends that routine screening for diabetes begin at age 45 in whites with no other risk factors for diabetes, and further recommends repeat testing for this group every

3 years thereafter if the results are within the normal range. The ADA recommends beginning surveillance at an earlier age, with more frequent monitoring, for individuals with any of the following risk factors for diabetes and cardiovascular disease: obesity, a first-degree relative with diabetes, membership in a high-risk ethnic population (African Americans; Hispanic Americans; Asian Americans, including Indian Asians; Pacific Islanders; and Native Americans), previous diagnosis of gestational diabetes or delivery of a baby larger than 9 pounds (44.1 kg), hypertension (>140/90 mm Hg), a high-density lipoprotein level ≤35 mg/dL, triglyceride level ≥250 mg/dL, or previous diagnosis of impaired fasting glucose (fasting plasma glucose level ≥110 mg/dL but <126 mg/dL) or impaired glucose tolerance (OGTT revealing 2-hour postload glucose level of ≥140 mg/dL but <200 mg/dL) (Expert Committee on the Diagnosis and Classification of Diabetes Mellitus 2000).

Because schizophrenia is associated with increased rates of diabetes mellitus or impaired glucose regulation, and because the newer, atypical antipsychotic agents appear to increase this risk even further, it seems reasonable that patients with schizophrenia, and especially patients taking atypical antipsychotic medications, should be screened for hyperglycemia before age 45 and monitored more frequently than every 3 years. This is especially appropriate in light of case reports of new-onset diabetes mellitus associated with atypical antipsychotic therapy in patients under 20 years of age. In addition, patients with higher risk factors should be examined more closely. African American, Asian, and Latino patients should be monitored closely, particularly if they have other risk factors for diabetes independent of ethnicity. If factors such as weight gain, elevated lipids, or hypertension develop, early interventions are necessary to prevent the onset of diabetes. Although we know very little about the underlying reasons that some patients treated with atypical antipsychotic agents experience DKA, undertaking a risk assessment with each patient may help in the selection of safer agents for each particular patient. We recommend monitoring weight changes and blood pressure at each office visit along with fasting glucose and lipids at baseline and every 3 months. Also, patients must be instructed to notify the treatment team if they experience any physical symptoms or medical disorders, because a number of DKA episodes have occurred in conjunction with other acute medical disorders, such as infections and pancreatitis. Finally, patients treated with atypical antipsychotic agents, particularly clozapine and olanzapine, should be screened more frequently.

Although data from published reports and clinical experience imply a difference among the atypical antipsychotic agents' impacts on glucose metabolism, it is too early to rule out a class effect. Ziprasidone may offer significant advantages because it appears to be weight neutral (Allison et al. 1999); however, additional clinical experience is necessary with this agent before definitive conclusions can be reached. Therefore, a reasonable approach would be to take baseline measures (fasting blood glucose, lipids, weight, blood pressure) on all patients, and fasting glucose and lipids every 6 months if these can be obtained. Weight and blood pressure can be monitored more frequently in the office. Monitoring of glycohemoglobin may be useful in this population in cases where fasting glucose is difficult to obtain. However, glycohemoglobin monitoring may not be sensitive enough to detect lower levels of hyperglycemia, glycohemoglobin changes will lag 2 to 3 months behind changes in glucose homeostasis, and criteria for diagnosing diabetes on the basis of glycohemoglobin do not exist. Education and referral to weight reduction and exercise programs may play a significant preventive role. In addition, weight gain should initiate meaningful dietary intervention. Finally, the clinician should be alert to the possibility of DKA (Lebovitz 2001).

If a patient develops diabetes while receiving treatment with an atypical antipsychotic agent, consideration should be given to switching to another antipsychotic agent. Although DKA appears to be uncommon, it is of great concern in connection with the risk of death. Patients who experience an episode of DKA should be switched to a different antipsychotic agent that has a lower impact on glucose metabolism. Reports and clinical experience suggest that in a case of atypical antipsychotic agent–associated diabetes or DKA, discontinuation of the antipsychotic agent may result in complete resolution of the hyperglycemia and diabetes. Clozapine-treated patients have few options. Clozapine remains the most effective agent for the treatment-resistant schizophrenia population, and patients often have failed to benefit from several other antipsychotic agents. Interventions to reduce the factors that contribute to impaired glucose intolerance, such as weight loss programs, encouraging exercise, and lowering the clozapine dose, may lead to improvement. For patients treated with other atypical agents, consideration for switching to another agent should be given in addition to the preceding interventions. Finally, diabetic patients who are placed on these agents must be monitored more closely to prevent a worsening in the control of serum glucose.

Conclusion

Atypical antipsychotic medications have helped to improve the lives of patients with schizophrenia by alleviating positive and negative symptoms and bringing some improvement in cognitive function. This improvement in cognitive function is helping patients to function in the home and in the workplace, thus improving the quality of patients' lives. However, the atypical antipsychotics appear to be associated with the development of glucose intolerance, new-onset diabetes mellitus, DKA, and exacerbation of existing diabetes mellitus. These disturbances in glucose metabolism have their own medical consequences, including cardiovascular disease, cerebrovascular disease, diabetic retinopathy, neuropathy, and diabetic nephropathy, all of which can lead to considerable morbidity and mortality. Thus, to minimize morbidity and mortality associated with the use of the atypical antipsychotic medications, close screening and monitoring for diabetes mellitus should become a priority for all clinicians treating schizophrenia patients receiving atypical antipsychotic therapy.

References

Allison DB, Mentore JL, Heo M, et al: Antipsychotic-induced weight gain: a comprehensive research synthesis. Am J Psychiatry 156:1686–1696, 1999

American Diabetes Association: Screening for type 2 diabetes. Diabetes Care 23 (suppl 1):S20–S23, 2000

Braceland FJ, Meduna LJ, Vaichulis JA: Delayed action of insulin in schizophrenia. Am J Psychiatry 102:108–110, 1945

Brambilla F, Guastalla A, Guerrini A, et al: Glucose-insulin metabolism in chronic schizophrenia. Dis Nerv Syst 37:98–103, 1976

Csernansky JG, Mahmoud R, Brenner R: A comparison of risperidone and haloperidol for the prevention of relapse in patients with schizophrenia. N Engl J Med 346:16–22, 2002

Dwyer DS, Liu Y, Bradley RJ: Dopamine receptor antagonists modulate glucose uptake in rat pheochromocytoma (PC12) cells. Neurosci Lett 274:151–154, 1999

Expert Committee on the Diagnosis and Classification of Diabetes Mellitus: Report of the Expert Committee on the Diagnosis and Classification of Diabetes Mellitus. Diabetes Care 23 (suppl 1):S4–S19, 2000

Fertig MK, Brooks VG, Shelton PS, et al: Hyperglycemia associated with olanzapine. J Clin Psychiatry 59:687–689, 1998

Fryburg D, O'Sullivan R, Siu C, et al: Insulin resistance in olanzapine- and ziprasidone-treated patients: interim results of a double blind controlled 6-week trial. Poster presented at the 39th annual meeting of the American College of Neuropsychopharmacology; San Juan, Puerto Rico, December 10–14, 2000

Gatta B, Rigalleau V, Gin H: Diabetic ketoacidosis with olanzapine treatment. Diabetes Care 22:1002–1003, 1999

Gerstein HC, Pais P, Pogue J, et al: Relationship of glucose and insulin levels to the risk of myocardial infarction: a case-control study. J Am Coll Cardiol 33:612–619, 1999

Goldstein LE, Sporn J, Brown S, et al: New-onset diabetes mellitus and diabetic ketoacidosis associated with olanzapine treatment. Psychosomatics 40:438–443, 1999

Griffiths J, Springuel P: Atypical antipsychotics: impaired glucose metabolism. Canadian Adverse Drug Reaction Newsletter 165:943–945, 947–949, 2001

Hagg S, Joelsson L, Mjorndal T, et al: Prevalence of diabetes and impaired glucose tolerance in patients with clozapine compared with patients treated with conventional depot neuroleptic medications. J Clin Psychiatry 59:294–299, 1998

Haupt DW, Newcomer JW: Hyperglycemia and antipsychotic medications. J Clin Psychiatry 62 (suppl 27):15–26, 2001

Henderson DC: Clinical experience with insulin resistance, diabetic ketoacidosis, and type 2 diabetes mellitus in patients treated with atypical antipsychotic agents. J Clin Psychiatry 62 (suppl 27):10–14, 2001a

Henderson DC: Atypical antipsychotic-induced diabetes mellitus: how strong is the evidence? CNS Drugs 16:1–13, 2001b

Henderson DC, Cagliero E, Gray C, et al: Clozapine, diabetes mellitus, weight gain, and lipid abnormalities: a five-year naturalistic study. Am J Psychiatry 157:975–981, 2000a

Henderson DC, Cagliero E, Borba CP, et al: Atypical antipsychotic agents and glucose metabolism: Bergman's MINMOD Analysis. Paper presented at the 40th annual meeting of the New Clinical Drug Evaluation Unit, Boca Raton, FL, May 30–June 2, 2000b

Isojarvi JI, Laatikainen TJ, Pakarinen AJ, et al: Polycystic ovaries and hyperandrogenism in women taking valproate for epilepsy. N Engl J Med 329:1383–1388, 1993

Isojarvi J, Rattya J, Myllyla VV, et al: Valproate, lamotrigine, and insulin-mediated risks in women with epilepsy. Ann Neurol 43:446–451, 1998

Kane J, Honigfeld G, Singer S, et al: Clozapine for the treatment-resistant schizophrenia: a double-blind comparison with chlorpromazine. Arch Gen Psychiatry 45:789–796, 1988

Koller EA, Doraiswamy PM: Olanzapine-associated diabetes mellitus. Pharmacotherapy 22:841–852, 2002

Koller E, Schneider B, Bennett K, et al: Clozapine-associated diabetes. Am J Med 111:716–723, 2001

Lebovitz HE: Diabetes: diagnosis, classification, and pathogenesis. J Clin Psychiatry 62 (suppl 27):5–9, 2001

Lindenmayer JP, Patel R: Olanzapine-induced ketoacidosis with diabetes mellitus [letter]. Am J Psychiatry 156:1471, 1999

Marinow A: Diabetes in chronic schizophrenia. Dis Nerv Syst 32:777–778, 1971

Melkersson KI, Hulting AL, Brismar KE: Different influences of classical antipsychotics and clozapine on glucose-insulin homeostasis in patients with schizophrenia or related psychoses. J Clin Psychiatry 60:783–791, 1999

Melkersson KI, Hulting AL, Brismar KE: Elevated levels of insulin, leptin, and blood lipids in olanzapine-treated patients with schizophrenia or related psychoses. J Clin Psychiatry 61:742–749, 2000

Meltzer HY: Putting metabolic side effects into perspective: risks versus benefits of atypical antipsychotics. J Clin Psychiatry 62 (suppl 27):35–39, 2001

Meltzer HY, Burnett S, Bastani B, et al: Effect of six months of clozapine treatment on the quality of life of chronic schizophrenic patients. Hosp Community Psychiatry 41:892–897, 1990

Meyer JM: Effects of atypical antipsychotics on weight and serum lipid levels. J Clin Psychiatry 62 (suppl 27):27–34, 2001

Mir S, Taylor D: Atypical antipsychotics and hyperglycaemia. Int Clin Psychopharmacol 16:63–73, 2001

Mukherjee S, Decina P, Bocola V, et al: Diabetes mellitus in schizophrenic patients. Compr Psychiatry 37:68–73, 1996

Newcomer JW: Introduction: metabolic disturbances associated with antipsychotic use. J Clin Psychiatry 62 (suppl 27):3–4, 2001

Pi-Snyder F: Medical hazards of obesity. Ann Intern Med 119:655–660, 1993

Popli A, Konicki P, Jurjus G, et al: Clozapine and associated diabetes mellitus. J Clin Psychiatry 58:108–111, 1997

Schwartz L, Munoz R: Blood sugar levels in patients treated with chlorpromazine. Am J Psychiatry 125:253–255, 1968

Selke G, Fucetola R, Cooper BP, et al: Atypical antipsychotic–induced differences in glucose regulation in schizophrenia independent of differences in adiposity (abstract). Abstr Soc Neurosci 26:275, 2000

Waitzkin L: A survey of unknown diabetes in a mental hospital, I. Diabetes 15:97–104, 1966a

Waitzkin L: A survey of unknown diabetics in a mental hospital, II: men from age fifty. Diabetes 15:164–172, 1966b

Westphal SA: The occurrence of diabetic ketoacidosis in non–insulin dependent diabetes and newly diagnosed diabetic adults. Am J Med 101:19–24, 1996

Wirshing DA, Spellberg BJ, Erhart SM, et al: Novel antipsychotics and new onset diabetes. Biol Psychiatry 44:778–783, 1998

Wirshing DA, Pierre JM, Eyeler J, et al: Risperidone-associated new-onset diabetes. Biol Psychiatry 50:148–149, 2001

Chapter 7

HIV and Hepatitis C in Patients With Schizophrenia

Milton L. Wainberg, M.D.
Francine Cournos, M.D.
Karen McKinnon, M.A.
Alan Berkman, M.D.

Introduction

Among the chronic health conditions experienced by people with schizophrenia, infection with human immunodeficiency virus (HIV) or hepatitis C virus (HCV) occurs with notable frequency. People who contract HIV face chronic illness, the likelihood of premature death, complicated medication regimens, barriers to medical care, and the neuropsychiatric sequelae of HIV infection itself. HCV is emerging as a significant public health issue due to the persistence of viremia in over 75% of infected persons, with resultant cirrhosis in up to 20% after 10 to 30 years and, in rare cases, hepatocellular carcinoma. It is estimated that in the United States less than 30% of people with HCV know they are infected (National Institutes of Health Consensus Development Conference Panel 1997).

Published rates of HIV infection among psychiatric patients are 3.1% to 23.9%, at least eight times higher than estimates for the general population (Cournos and McKinnon 1997; Rosenberg et al. 2001). These seroprevalence studies were all conducted on the East Coast; in other parts of the United States, no published seroprevalence studies exist to shed light on whether people with severe mental illness in those localities are at increased risk of HIV infection. HIV infection rates among patients with schizophrenia rarely have been differentiated from rates among others with psychotic disorders; but when they have, no significant differences emerged, countering expectations that infection rates might be lower among those with schizophrenia than among those with other severe mental illnesses.

Rates of HCV infection among people with schizophrenia have received far less attention. A large retrospective Italian study found that 6.7% of 1,180 patients hospitalized for mental retardation, psychosis, and dementia were infected with HCV (Cividini et al. 1997). Psychosis and a history of trauma were statistically significant independent risk factors associated with HCV infection (Cividini et al. 1997). In the United States, the magnitude of the threat has been quantified in one published study that found a prevalence of 19.6% among 751 psychiatric inpatients and outpatients tested in a multisite study on the East Coast (Rosenberg et al. 2001). On the West Coast, preliminary findings among 508 state hospital adult inpatients show that 20.3% were HCV seropositive (Meyer, in press). These rates contrast with the general population rate of approximately 1.8%.

Psychiatric symptoms and disabilities differentiate this population from others and may increase HIV/HCV risk among people with the most serious psychiatric disorders, either by directly affecting behavior or by interfering with the ability to acquire or use information about these illnesses to practice safer behaviors. Wherever they work, psychiatrists and other mental health care providers often are in the best position to enhance their patients' skills in modifying high-risk behaviors and to connect infected psychiatric patients with the HIV- and HCV-related services they need.

Sexual Risk Behaviors Among People With Schizophrenia and Their Association With Psychiatric and Situational Factors

Most studies of sexual risk behavior among people with psychiatric disorders have not linked behaviors to biological outcomes, but risk for HIV transmission is potentially very high; the role of sexual transmission in HCV infection is weak and poorly understood even in the general population.

Sexual risk behaviors among people in psychiatric treatment are common, with interview studies in Brazil, Canada, Spain, and the United States revealing that a majority of patients were sexually active with a partner in the past year (Acuda and Sebit 1996; Carey et al. 1997; Chuang and Atkinson 1996; Oliveira 1997). Moreover, reports of multiple sex partners are common among sexually active psychiatric patients (Chuang and Atkinson 1996). The sexual activity of people with serious mental illness also is characterized by a lack of condom use in a majority of sexual occasions, a finding true for both men and women (Carey et al. 1997; Cournos et al. 1993; Hanson et al. 1992).

Few studies have differentiated risks by psychiatric diagnosis, so critical information is lacking about patients with schizophrenia-spectrum illnesses; however, data on diagnostic and symptom contributions to sexual risk behavior are beginning to appear. Being sexually active has been found to be associated with a diagnosis of schizophrenia but not with bipolar disorder. Trading sex for money or drugs was more than three times as likely among patients with schizophrenia than among those with other diagnoses, and more than five times as likely among those with certain positive symptoms such as delusions (McKinnon et al. 1996).

Situational factors also appear to contribute to sexual risk taking. Extended periods of institutionalization in same-sex units in hospitals, shelters, or prisons may foster high-risk same-sex activity, often among those who do not identify themselves as gay or lesbian. This behavior is particularly risky for men. One study that directly compared psychiatric patients with nonpsychiatric groups found that psychiatric patients are more likely to engage in same-sex activity (McDermott et al. 1994).

The best predictor of condom use is having a condom. Institutional obstacles to condom acquisition are another factor likely to impede patients' initiative and ability to practice safer sex. Making condoms anonymously available to all patients, including inpatients with off-ward privileges or who engage in consensual sex on the ward, has been shown to be a cost-effective primary prevention intervention (Carmen and Brady 1990). Sexual victimization, in which there is increased likelihood of unprotected intercourse (Herbert 1995), also has been widely reported by psychiatric inpatients (Goodman and Fallot 1998). Among outpatients, one in eight reported having been pressured, coerced, or forced into unwanted sex in the past year (Carey et al. 1997). Identification of patients in abusive relationships will facilitate their engagement in individual and group interventions to help them practice assertive behaviors and negotiating skills to increase self-protective behaviors, including condom use.

Recurrent institutionalization, homelessness, transient living circumstances, alienation from supportive social relationships, and lack of pri-
vacy can all interrupt long-term relationships, reinforcing the tendency to
have unfamiliar partners. Studies report that 10% to 16% of psychiatric patients had sex in the past year with someone they had known less than 24
hours (Chuang and Atkinson 1996; Kalichman et al. 1994; Kelly et al.
1992). These conditions also may make changing risk behaviors difficult
for people with serious mental illness or may limit sexual opportunities to
those that confer greater risk. Unemployment also may contribute to
greater sexual risk taking (Acuda and Sebit 1996), possibly through pres-
sures toward engaging in survival sex or commercial sex work.

Having a sexually transmitted disease (STD) also renders a person biologically more vulnerable to acquiring subsequent infections when exposed. Between 9% and 36% of psychiatric inpatients and outpatients are
diagnosed with one or more STDs at some time in their lives (Carey et al.
1997; Rosenberg et al. 2001). Moreover, a patient may have an STD without being aware of it, and will likely remain untreated unless screening for
STDs is included with other prevention efforts aimed at risk behaviors for
sexually transmitted infections.

Substance Use Risk Behaviors Among People With Schizophrenia and Their Association With Psychiatric and Situational Factors

In the United States, psychiatric patients with identified comorbid alcohol
or other drug use disorders have a significantly higher rate of HIV infection
than those without (McKinnon and Cournos 1998), even if they have never
injected drugs. In this population, any lifetime instance of drug injection or
needle sharing appears to increase the risk of being HIV infected more
than sixfold (Ayuso-Mateos et al. 1997; Horwath et al. 1996; Rosenberg et
al. 2001). Similar to the case for the general population, HCV infection in
psychiatric patients is most strongly associated with injection drug use, and
to a lesser extent with other drug use and poverty. Of 122 patients identified with HCV in Rosenberg's study, 91 were injection drug users, 21 reported sniffing cocaine, 17 had used crack, and 24 had used both types of
cocaine, with only 7 reporting no drug-related risks (Rosenberg et al. 2001).

A history of drug injection has been noted among 1% to 26% of psychiatric patients (Carey et al. 1997; Rosenberg et al. 2001; Susser et al. 1996),

and 5% to 12% report having ever shared needles or other injection paraphernalia (Carey et al. 1997; Rosenberg et al. 2001). Moreover, psychiatric patients who inject tend to do so intermittently rather than regularly, so drug injection histories often are overlooked in mental health settings. In a group of chronically ill psychiatric patients, drug injection was not predicted by psychiatric diagnosis, chronicity, level of functioning, or psychiatric symptoms (Horwath et al. 1996). In another study, drug injection was significantly more common among those with depressive disorder than among those with schizophrenia, and patients with bipolar disorder had the lowest rates of all (McDermott et al. 1994). As in the general population, alcohol or other drugs often are part of psychiatric patients' sexual experience and may decrease the motivation or ability to have protected sex. Fifteen percent to 45% of psychiatric inpatients and outpatients reported using substances during sex in the past year (Carey et al. 1997; Chuang and Atkinson 1996; Katz et al. 1994; Menon and Pomerantz 1997), with comparable rates seen in men and women.

HIV/HCV Knowledge Among People With Severe Mental Illness and Their Providers

AIDS is the ultimate result of HIV infection, and knowledge about AIDS-related issues among United States and Canadian psychiatric patients appears to be relatively good compared with that of nonpsychiatric groups. Correct responses to AIDS knowledge questionnaires in a variety of psychiatric patient groups ranged from 63% to 80% (Chuang and Atkinson 1996; McKinnon et al. 1996; Otto-Salaj et al. 1998), a comparable accuracy rate to that found in the general United States population (Hardy 1990). Still, many psychiatric patients held critical misinterpretations. For example, in one study 42% were unaware they could be infected by injection drug use (Katz et al. 1994), and in another, 48% believed that careful cleansing after sex would provide protection from the virus (Otto-Salaj et al. 1998). Comparable studies about HCV knowledge among patients have not been completed. Although knowledge is necessary, it is not sufficient to reduce unsafe behaviors.

Preliminary findings from qualitative interviews with medical and mental health care providers show widespread consensus that HCV is a major public healthcare issue (P. Mendel and G. Ryan, unpublished data, February 2002). Interviews with providers at 32 agencies in New York City and Los Angeles showed adequate knowledge about how to identify HCV-antibody-positive clients, at least among agencies with established medical services. In general, testing for HCV is less burdensome because it does not involve the counseling, confidentiality, or stigma issues usually associated with HIV testing; yet there is great variation among providers on how to proceed once HCV-positive patients are identified. Uncertainty about the efficacy of current treatments, exclusion/inclusion criteria for treatment, and the division of responsibility among medical specialties for managing treatment are paramount concerns.

Mendel and Ryan's qualitative data suggest that, in practice, many mental health care providers are unsure of how many of their clients have HCV, except for a general sense that the numbers are increasing. Staff in mental health agencies were more concerned with diabetes and tuberculosis (because of the difficulty in daily self-management and the risk of contagion, respectively) than with either HCV or HIV. In addition, these qualitative data show that mental health and substance abuse treatment providers were generally unaware of the depressive side effects of interferon therapy, with only two agencies in New York City recounting specific in-service trainings that covered HCV along with other diseases. We believe that improved HCV screening followed by referral for evaluation of every HCV-positive patient, including those with schizophrenia, whose psychiatric condition is stable is now warranted.

Basic Overview of Course of Illness and Treatment of HIV/AIDS

Approximately 940,000 persons in North America and about 40 million persons worldwide are infected with HIV. Infection with HIV is a chronic disease that normally runs its course over many years. AIDS is a late-stage manifestation of HIV infection, characterized by increasing viral load of HIV in the blood and declining immune function (as measured by CD4 T cell counts), leading to a broad spectrum of diseases. According to the definition of the Centers for Disease Control and Prevention (CDC), the diagnosis of AIDS is made in an HIV-positive individual who has at least one of 25 AIDS-defining conditions (e.g., *Pneumocystis carinii* pneumonia [PCP] or HIV-associated dementia [HAD]) or a CD4 T cell count lower than 200 cells per cubic millimeter. The human immunodeficiency virus has been clearly identified as the cause of AIDS (Barre-Sinoussi et al. 1983; Gallo et al. 1984). This virus invades the nervous system, causes persistent viremia, and weakens the humoral and cellular immune response of most infected people. HIV has a remarkably complex viral genome, which probably underlies its profound pathogenicity (Varmus 1988).

First identified in 1983, HIV contains ribonucleic acid (RNA) as its genetic material, as well as the enzyme reverse transcriptase, which is required to translate viral RNA into deoxyribonucleic acid (DNA) so that it can use the host cell's nucleic material to replicate. The replicated virus particles, initially strung together, must be split apart by the protease enzyme before they are extruded from the host cell in order for them to become functional and damaging to the immune system. HIV mutates rapidly, making drug resistance a major problem and contributing to the difficulties in producing an effective vaccine. HIV-1 is the form of the virus that is the causative agent of disease in the United States and much of the rest of the world, but another strain, HIV-2, occurs in West Africa, with scattered cases appearing recently in Asia. HIV-2 is associated with considerably slower disease progression than HIV-1. Having either virus does not alter the vulnerability for infection with or confer humoral protection to the other strain (Warner 1997). Some experts estimate that efforts to develop an effective HIV vaccine may be successful within the next 5 to 10 years.

HIV Transmissibility

Although HIV has been isolated from a variety of body fluids, including blood, semen, vaginal secretions, breast milk, urine, saliva, and tears, the risk of transmission is a consequence of the amount of virus present and the type of exposure to infected bodily fluids. HIV is found in such small quantities in tears, saliva, and urine that casual contact with these fluids is a theoretically possible but very unlikely mode of transmission. Epidemiological studies indicate that semen, cervical and vaginal secretions, breast milk, and blood and blood products are the predominant, if not exclusive, vehicles for viral transmission (Staprans and Feinberg 1997). Although uncommon, infection is possible through the exposure of cuts in skin or mucous membranes to HIV-infected blood.

HIV is typically spread by sexual contact, exposure to infected blood (transfusions, blood products, percutaneous or intravenous injections with contaminated syringes or needles, etc.) and through perinatal transmission from mother to child (Warner 1997). Penile–vaginal and penile–anal intercourse are considered the highest-risk sexual behaviors, in addition to activities that cause a rupture of tissue and the presence of blood. Although the risk of infection is somewhat higher for the recipient of semen than for the insertive partner, transmission has been documented in both directions. Because HIV is present in vaginal secretions, preseminal fluid, and semen, oral sex has also been documented as a mode of transmission for the recipient of fluids, as has the sharing of sexual toys, although to a lesser extent. Certain cofactors enhance the risk of sexual transmission of HIV, including the presence of sexually transmitted infections such as syphilis and chlamydia, and genital lesions or genital or mucous membrane bruising during sexual activity.

Sharing needles or other equipment during injection is a very efficient means of transmitting HIV and amounts to a direct inoculation of viral particles from the infected to the noninfected person. As with other routes of transmission, the likelihood of transmission increases with the size of the viral inoculum. Even noninjection substance use may increase the risk for HIV by increasing the chance that an individual will engage in high-risk behaviors due to lowered sexual inhibitions, impaired judgment, increased impulsiveness, or the exchange of sex for drugs or money to buy drugs. Transfusion with infected blood and the use of infected blood products almost always results in acquisition of HIV, although testing of donated blood and blood products has practically eliminated the chances of this occurrence in the industrialized countries.

HIV Testing

The most commonly used HIV test—enzyme-linked immunosorbent assay (ELISA) followed, if positive, by Western blot—detects the presence of antibodies produced by the host as an immune response to certain genetic components of the virus, but not the presence of the virus itself. Although sensitive and specific, these tests can give false negative or indeterminate results, especially early in the course of infection. False positive results may occur as well, which is why blanket testing is problematic when carried out in a population in which the prevalence of HIV infection is very low. There is a period following initial infection and before antibody development when an individual is infectious but has negative ELISA and Western blot test results. The current generation of ELISA tests has reduced this "window period" to 3 or 4 weeks in most patients, but an occasional individual may take months to develop a positive test result (Corbitt et al. 1991). However, direct measurement of viral presence using the polymerase chain reaction (PCR) assay will usually show extremely high levels of virus during this window period.

Viral Load and Resistance Assays

Viral load, a quantifiable measurement of how many viral particles are present in a cubic centimeter of blood, can be determined by several different assays, some of which detect as few as 50 viral particles per cubic centimeter of blood. Below that threshold of measurement, the result is reported as "nondetectable." This does not indicate that there is no virus present in blood at all, nor does it measure the amount of virus in lymphoid tissue or in the central nervous system (CNS). Viral load is a strong predictor of disease progression in untreated patients. For those on antiretroviral therapy, CD4 T cell counts are the stronger predictor of clinical outcome and are useful in monitoring clinical response to therapy (O'Brien et al. 1996). Predicting responses to antiviral medications can be accomplished by testing for drug resistance, a problem increasingly seen in clinical practice. Resistance assays fall into two classes: genotyping examines the virus for mutations known to confer drug resistance, whereas phenotyping tests the susceptibility of the patient's virus to specific medications.

Natural History of HIV Disease

HIV targets host CD4 T lymphocytes by identifying certain surface molecules and attaching to and entering the cells (Staprans and Feinberg 1997). This begins the process of using the viral reverse transcriptase enzyme to transcribe viral RNA to DNA, which allows the virus to use the host cell's machinery to make new whole viral particles, called virions. These virions spread rapidly to uninfected lymphocytes, where they replicate more copies of HIV. As the host produces circulating antibodies against HIV, the host is said to seroconvert. Although the immune system may initially contain the infection, the course is set for chronic persistent viral replication. Without treatment, eventually there is near complete destruction of the CD4 T lymphocyte population in the vast majority of infected people. Current knowledge suggests that a person's initial viral "setpoint," the capacity of his or her immune system to limit viral replication, is the strongest predictor of untreated disease progression (Mellors et al. 1996).

The range and severity of symptoms in primary HIV infection varies considerably, with an acute 1-month mononucleosis-like viral syndrome developing in about 40%–60% of patients (Levy 1993). Symptoms can include fever, headache, lymphadenopathy, malaise, myalgia, rash, stiff neck, and other meningeal signs and symptoms, accompanied by transient intense viremia and an acute fall in CD4 T cell count in the peripheral blood from its normal range of 800–1,200 cells per cubic millimeter (Staprans and Feinberg 1997). The more severe this syndrome is, the more likely that the untreated patient will progress rapidly to AIDS (Keet et al. 1993). Clinicians are now hoping to slow down progression to AIDS by initiating highly active antiretroviral treatment (HAART) during primary infection, and recent evidence suggests that such treatment may provide a unique window for enhancing the body's own immune response to HIV. However, primary infection often goes undetected and HAART requires long-term near-perfect adherence with multiple drugs taken several times daily.

Once the symptoms of primary infection subside and an antiviral immune response appears, patients usually enter a chronic, clinically asymptomatic or minimally symptomatic state despite continuous active viral replication. This period may last only a few years in some infected individuals, but the majority of HIV-positive patients develop overt immunodeficiency in approximately 10 years, with a small cohort demonstrating sustained long-term (>10 years) symptom-free HIV infection (Lifson et al. 1991; Staprans and Feinberg 1997). During chronic infection, the development of symptoms, a low CD4 cell count, and a high viral load should initiate a discussion between clinician and patient about antiretroviral treatment. The patient's ability to adhere to the regimen is, of course, pivotal to the decision.

The spectrum of HIV-associated illnesses that eventually develops includes constitutional symptoms (e.g., weight loss, fatigue, fever, night sweats) and involvement of multiple organ systems. Opportunistic infections (OIs) are multiple and can occur throughout the body. These include fungal infections (e.g., oral or esophageal candidiasis [thrush]), PCP, and mycobacterial infections (e.g., tuberculosis and *Mycobacterium avium* complex). Cancers, such as Kaposi's sarcoma and lymphoma, are other manifestations of severe immunosuppression. Prophylactic regimens can reduce the occurrence of many OIs in immunocompromised patients.

Neuropsychiatric Manifestations

HIV infection presents a spectrum of neuropsychiatric sequelae that can pose diagnostic and treatment quandaries to clinicians. In patients with serious and persistent psychiatric illness, some of the early, subtle neuropsychiatric symptoms may be difficult to differentiate from preexisting symptoms of their psychiatric illness. HIV is neurotropic (O'Brien 1994), enters the CNS soon after infection (Resnick et al. 1988), and can acutely induce headache and meningeal signs as already noted. Long-term clinical sequelae of CNS infection range from subtle neurocognitive impairment to frank dementia, and their incidence increases with HIV illness progression. OIs and neoplasms that follow immunosuppression can also affect the CNS, resulting in mood disorders, psychosis, cognitive disorders, delirium, and other neuropsychiatric abnormalities. In addition, prescribed and recreational psychoactive substance use may create neuropsychiatric complications, and must be considered in the differential diagnosis of patients who present with new mental status changes (McDaniel et al. 1997).

HIV-related neurocognitive disorders are diagnoses of exclusion made after other etiologies have been ruled out through a comprehensive evaluation. Common cognitive disorders in HIV infection include minor cognitive–motor disorder (MCMD) and HAD. MCMD is a mild syndrome of motor and/or cognitive dysfunction with minimal impairment in functioning (McDaniel et al. 1997) and is characterized by at least two of the following features: impaired attention or concentration, mental slowing, impaired memory, slowed movements, impaired coordination, personality change, irritability, and lability. MCMD does not necessarily progress to the more severe disorder of HAD (Masliah et al. 1996).

HAD is a subcortical dementia, and criteria for its diagnosis include acquired abnormality in two or more cognitive domains causing functional impairment; acquired abnormality in motor performance or decline in motivation or emotional control; no clouding of consciousness (delirium); and no confounding etiology. Although the exact pathophysiology of HAD remains unclear, HAD is relatively common, particularly in more advanced stages of HIV infection (McDaniel et al. 1997). Patients may also have neuropsychiatric impairments verifiable by testing that do not meet criteria for MCMD or HAD but that may result in functional impairment.

Psychiatric symptoms due to HIV-related medical conditions tend to occur in advanced stages of illness with significant evidence of immunosuppression and CD4 cell counts below 200 (American Psychiatric Association 2000). Therefore, among patients with advanced HIV disease who have a preexisting severe mental illness, psychiatric changes should not be attributed to a relapse until a complete medical workup has ruled out other causes. Mental status changes due to a medical etiology can include shifts in level of consciousness characteristic of delirium, cognitive impairment, mood changes, and psychotic symptoms. The differential diagnosis (Wainberg et al. 2000) includes not only the neuropsychiatric manifestations of HIV itself but also OIs (toxoplasmosis, cryptococcus, tuberculous meningitis), lymphoma, and delirium from metabolic derangement, substance use, or drug toxicity (McDaniel et al. 1997).

HIV/AIDS Treatment

Clinical management is intended to decrease viral load, increase CD4 cell count, provide prophylaxis against OIs as appropriate, treat OIs when present, and decrease morbidity and mortality. New knowledge about the life cycle of HIV and the advent of different classes of antiretroviral medications have altered the state-of-the-art of treatment, which now requires combination antiretroviral therapies and the prophylaxis of OIs according to guidelines based on the prevalence of each OI at various stages of immunodeficiency. Except in cases of HIV primary infection, pregnancy in an HIV-infected woman, or symptomatic HIV disease, antiretroviral therapy in asymptomatic patients known to be HIV positive is usually initiated when the CD4 cell count is between 200 and 350.

Part of instituting antiretroviral therapy involves ensuring that patients recognize their HIV infection, have access to health care, develop ongoing provider relationships, and are motivated to adhere to complicated treatments, even during an asymptomatic phase of infection. Taking a combination of at least three antiretroviral medications is currently the best way to accomplish this objective. If a patient is not ready to adhere to antiretroviral therapy (e.g., because of chaotic life due to psychiatric instability, substance use, and/or homelessness; lack of motivation; or insufficient social supports), it is important to first address barriers to adherence. Evidence demonstrates that 95% adherence is necessary to suppress fully the replication of virus that is sensitive to the regimen being administered. Even though 80%–95% adherence decreases morbidity and mortality, long-term implications are unclear (e.g., resistant strains, neuropsychiatric sequelae). Mental health professionals often have important roles in promoting adherence.

Antiretroviral therapies are classified according to the specific step inhibited in the HIV life cycle within the CD4 lymphocyte. Individually, these agents are not very potent in inhibiting viral replication, but combining classes enables different replication steps to be "attacked," enhancing the possibility of interrupting viral reproduction. The four major classes of therapies currently available are 1) nucleoside reverse transcriptase inhibitors (NRTIs), which act by incorporating themselves into the DNA of the virus through the reverse transcriptase enzyme, resulting in DNA that is incomplete and incapable of creating new virus (didanosine, lamivudine, stavudine, zalcitabine, zidovudine [AZT], abacavir); 2) nonnucleoside reverse transcriptase inhibitors (NNRTIs), which stop HIV production by binding directly to reverse transcriptase and preventing the conversion of viral RNA to DNA (delavirdine, efavirenz, nevirapine); 3) nucleotide reverse transcriptase inhibitors, which have a mechanism of action similar to that of NRTIs (tenofovir); and 4) protease inhibitors (PIs), which affect the last stage of viral reproduction by inhibiting the viral protease enzyme from cleaving the viral protein chains into smaller infectious virions (amprenavir, indinavir, lopinavir/ritonavir, nelfinavir, ritonavir, saquinavir).

The PIs are often potent inhibitors of one or more cytochrome P450 enzymes, which may have implications for interactions with psychiatric and other medications. A new category of antiretrovirals, called fusion inhibitors, is being developed and acts by inhibiting HIV from binding to CD4 cells.

Basic Overview of Course of Illness and Treatment of HCV

Approximately 4 million persons in the United States and probably more than 100 million persons worldwide are infected with HCV. The virus has the unique ability to cause persistent infection in a majority of infected people. The immunological correlates of protection and viral clearance and the pathogenesis of liver injury are yet to be defined, but recent studies suggest the importance of cell-mediated immune responses. Although a large proportion of infected persons become chronic carriers, most have relatively mild disease with slow progression. However, chronic and progressive HCV carries significant morbidity and mortality and is a major cause of cirrhosis, end-stage liver disease, and liver cancer. Development of an effective HCV vaccine is not imminent, but recent advances in technology and basic knowledge of molecular virology and immunology may engender novel approaches to the fundamental problems encountered in vaccine development. Vaccines continue to be pursued, since current therapy for HCV is poorly tolerated and not effective for a substantial number of patients.

HCV Transmission and Testing

Given preliminary estimates that one in five patients with severe mental illness is infected with HCV, a strong argument can be made that all such persons should be screened for the virus. Certainly, all patients known to be infected with HIV should be screened for anti-HCV antibodies as part of their initial evaluation, as should those with high-risk behavior. HCV is primarily spread through infected blood and is therefore a common complication of injection drug use. HCV may be spread by maternal fetal transmission and by noninjected drug use activities as well. Risk for sexual transmission is low but not absent. In a significant minority of cases the mode of transmission is unknown. Like HIV, rates of HCV in the United States are higher in African Americans and Latinos than among Caucasians.

HCV infection should be confirmed with qualitative PCR assay if the patient is at low risk and the diagnosis seems in doubt. Moreover, there is a small but measurable false negative rate for antibody testing in patients who are severely immunosuppressed.

Natural History of HCV Disease

Acute HCV disease is usually asymptomatic, but 25%–35% of patients develop some constitutional symptoms or jaundice. Serum alanine aminotransferase (ALT) levels frequently rise, fluctuate, and fall again, suggesting recovery from the acute phase. Following acute infection, however, HCV is not easily cleared by the immune system, and 75%–80% of acute HCV infections become chronic, as evidenced by persistent or intermittent HCV viremia.

Patients infected with HCV should be advised to minimize or preferably discontinue intake of alcohol. Chronic HCV infection can cause inflammatory infiltration, particularly of the portal tracts, as well as focal liver cell necrosis and fibrosis that bridges between portal tracts. Hepatitis C is the leading cause of liver transplantation in the United States. About 10%–20% of patients progress to cirrhosis within 20–30 years of infection, and among those with cirrhosis, 1%–4% per year will develop hepatocellular carcinoma.

Immunosuppression associated with HIV appears to significantly alter the natural history and clinical course of HCV, with HCV-associated cirrhosis occurring more frequently in patients with HCV–HIV co-infection (33%) than in HCV alone (11%). People with HCV do not tolerate HAART as well, which can interfere with effective HIV treatment. Data indicate that liver failure due to HCV is the leading non-AIDS cause of death in HIV-infected individuals (Community Research Initiative on AIDS 2000; Vento et al. 1998). All patients co-infected with HCV and HIV, or infected with either virus alone, should be screened for immunity to hepatitis A and B; and if not immune, they should be immunized with both hepatitis A vaccine and hepatitis B vaccine. Acute infection with hepatitis A virus, normally a relatively benign and self-limited disease, is more likely to result in fulminant hepatic necrosis in the presence of HCV infection or any other chronic liver disease (Vento et al. 1998). Hepatitis A vaccine is safe for HIV-infected patients, and more than two-thirds of HIV-infected patients immunized with hepatitis A vaccine develop a protective antibody response. Patients without antibody protection for hepatitis A and B viruses can receive a combined vaccine that confers protection against both viruses.

HCV Treatment

Diagnostic testing to determine the presence of HCV viremia and the extent of liver pathology should be completed as early as possible in the care of a patient infected with HCV. Liver biopsy is useful in evaluating liver damage and deciding type of treatment; elevation in serum transaminases in the absence of inflammation or fibrosis typically is not an indication for treatment. Patients with active HCV infection or evidence of chronic liver disease should be referred to a specialist with experience in treating hepatitis C for evaluation and guidance regarding possible treatment. Treatment recommendations should be individualized, and not all patients with HCV should receive treatment. Factors to be considered in the selection of patients for treatment include the patient's immune status; the presence of moderate to severe inflammation and/or fibrosis, which predicts the likelihood of progression to cirrhosis in the absence of treatment; the likelihood of a favorable response to therapy, which varies with HCV viral load (lower viral load predicts better response) and genotype; HIV viral load if co-infected; the patient's commitment to therapy; and the risk of adverse effects of treatment, particularly for those with underlying psychiatric illness (National Digestive Diseases Information Clearinghouse 2003). In those who are also HIV positive, antiretroviral therapy may need to be modified, delayed, or interrupted in order to complete an adequate course of therapy for HCV. The effectiveness of treatment is assessed by following HCV viral load.

The goal of HCV treatment is cure of the infection, manifested by reduction in hepatitis C viral load to undetectable, normalization of transaminase (ALT and aspartate transaminase [AST]), and cessation of liver disease progression. Combination therapy with daily, oral ribavirin and once-weekly subcutaneous peginterferon-alpha-2b given over 6 to 12 months (depending on genotype and response) is emerging as the standard therapy for HCV and is clearly indicated in patients 18 to 60 years of age who have persistently abnormal ALT levels, HCV RNA in serum, and evidence on liver biopsy of chronic hepatitis with either fibrosis or moderate degrees of inflammatory activity (National Institutes of Health Consensus Development Conference Panel 1997).

Psychiatric symptoms during interferon therapy for viral hepatitis have been a crucial concern in consultation-liaison psychiatry. Interferon and ribavirin have potential neuropsychiatric side effects, including apathy, cognitive changes, irritability, depression, and suicidal thoughts. However, there have been few studies of this problem, and those that exist are not focused on people with schizophrenia. Nonetheless, it is worth noting that at least one study of nonschizophrenic patients suggests that the risk of serious psychiatric symptoms during interferon-alpha treatment may not be high, and that psychiatric illness or the possibility of psychiatric complications should not be used as a reason to refuse this treatment to patients with hepatitis C (Mulder et al. 2000). Nevertheless, psychiatric disorders may influence the course of treatment of HCV infection, and clinicians as well as internists should be aware of the substantial psychiatric comorbidity in these patients. Although neuropsychiatric complications of HCV itself are not a significant problem, some of the symptoms of liver failure, such as fatigue, loss of appetite, loss of sexual drive, and impotence, can overlap with the complications of interferon treatment, the symptoms of psychiatric disorders, and the side effects of psychotropic drugs.

Clinical Considerations

Risk Reduction Interventions and Strategies for HIV/HCV

HIV prevention programs that primarily dispense AIDS information have not been shown to influence risk behavior levels because, as evidence from studies demonstrates, knowledge by itself is necessary but not sufficient to produce behavioral changes. Intensive, small-group programs that simultaneously target knowledge, attitudes, motivations, and cognitive and behavioral skills have been tried and found to produce reductions in high-risk sexual behaviors, including some that are substance related, among people with serious mental illness. Effective elements from randomized outcome trials of these HIV risk-reduction interventions (Kelly 1997; Otto-Salaj et al. 2001) include 1) information and skills training in sexual assertiveness, negotiation, problem solving, use of condoms, and risk self-management; 2) intensive sessions (6–15 hours to achieve reductions in high-risk behaviors); 3) training participants to become AIDS educators or advocates; 4) booster or maintenance sessions, which appear to be necessary to sustain safer behaviors; 5) gender sensitivity training employing single-gender groups for dealing with same-sex partner issues or for decreasing patients' anxiety about discussing sexual issues with the opposite sex, or mixed-gender groups for increasing generalization from group exercises to real-life situations for heterosexual patients; 6) inclusion of sexually abstinent patients to train those who may not remain abstinent or who may validate for other patients the legitimate choice of an abstinent lifestyle; and 7) harm reduction as the ultimate goal for both sexual and drug-related risk behaviors. Patients can benefit from participating in mixed–HIV serostatus prevention groups; no one need reveal their HIV status unless they wish to do so. Whatever the group's composition, group leaders should leave time at the end of each session to discuss patients' personal issues privately and to address their needs by making appropriate referrals, including ones to HIV test sites.

Because HCV shares modes of transmission with HIV, groups focused on HIV risk reduction may also wish to impart information about HCV and the possibility of acquiring HCV infection through high-risk behaviors. Prevention efforts aimed at HCV are essential for patients who are currently (or at risk for) injecting drugs, because injection drug use is the risk factor responsible for the majority of HCV cases.

Once staff have received training to perform prevention interventions, they typically become motivated to start intervention groups for patients. Keeping groups going can be difficult in programs that have little patient turnover; groups work best in day programs and outpatient programs. In inpatient units, short lengths of stay may limit the number of sessions patients can attend, but that should not discourage staff from setting up such programs.

In the case of HIV-positive patients, individual counseling can reinforce patients' motivations to protect themselves and others. Clinicians can encourage disclosure to sex partners and use of condoms. Fully informed decisions about risk and protection of others are the goals. Support groups also are effective at reducing the isolation many patients experience after receiving an HIV diagnosis.

Accessing the Range of HIV/HCV-Related Services That Psychiatric Patients Need

Mental health service settings vary in their ability to offer HIV-related interventions, and the range of services available may not yet be meeting the needs of people with severe mental illness (McKinnon et al. 1999). With respect to HCV, Mendel and Ryan's preliminary findings suggest that patients with these psychiatric disorders often are thought "not good candidates" for HCV treatment, with several HIV clinics implementing policies excluding patients with serious psychiatric histories from HCV treatment despite the lack of evidence to support their concerns about maintaining adherence or triggering a major psychiatric event. One medical director at a clinic in a large hospital was willing to engage severely mentally ill patients in HCV treatment, but only if they were under heavily supervised mental health care. Implementing such arrangements could be helpful in initiating treatment and conducting mental health evaluations of candidates already on HCV treatment.

People with serious mental illness usually can undergo HIV counseling and antibody testing without inordinate distress or worsening of their psychiatric symptoms (Oquendo and Tricarico 1996). Clinicians can use their clinical judgment to determine when a patient's psychiatric condition permits optimal coping with any result, although HIV testing often can proceed when a patient is in the hospital for treatment of an acute episode. In fact, appropriate testing of inpatients has some advantages if the entire process can be completed before hospital discharge. (This is more likely now that the newly approved rapid test is available.) In these cases, staff can ensure that patients receive posttest counseling and follow-up appointments and can address any worsening of the patient's psychiatric condition in the event of a distressing test result.

Clinicians have an important role in helping their patients understand the implications of either a negative or a positive HIV antibody test result. Involvement in pretest counseling can ensure that patients have the capacity to give consent to testing; prepare themselves for the stress related to waiting for the result and the consequences of learning it; and appropriately anticipate, prevent, or manage exacerbations of psychiatric symptoms.

Voluntary HIV testing is the norm for people with serious mental illness so that those who are HIV positive can seek treatment and change their risk behaviors and yet be protected against discrimination. The capacity to consent to testing hinges on the ability to understand the information being conveyed and to draw reasonable conclusions from it. People with serious mental illness are considered to have this capacity unless an assessment determines otherwise, in which case consent may be given by a person who is legally authorized to do so. Informed consent for HIV antibody testing should include an explanation of the test, its purpose, the meaning of the results, and the benefits of early diagnosis and medical intervention. In addition, explanation should be given of the voluntary nature of the test, the individual's right to withdraw consent at any time, the availability of anonymous testing, and confidentiality and the circumstances under which test results may be disclosed with or without the individual's agreement.

The first step in the HIV counseling and testing process is to obtain a risk history. Rather than asking, "Have you ever...?" asking "How often have you...?" is more likely to elicit useful risk information without raising a patient's defenses by implying that the clinician will judge such behaviors negatively or consider them unusual.

The point of the risk assessment is to elicit behaviorally specific information about patients' sexual behaviors and drug use. Most patients, when queried in a direct and nonjudgmental way, are cooperative and forthcoming. The ease the clinician demonstrates in discussing sex and drug use will set the anxiety level for the patient, and normalizing any patient discomfort can create a more relaxed tone.

Clinicians should ensure that patients are referred for HIV testing on a regular basis whenever a patient asks for it, and when a patient has current or past risk behaviors, is pregnant, has physical signs suggestive of HIV infection or AIDS, has psychiatric symptoms that suggest CNS dysfunction, or has a positive PPD (Mantoux) tuberculin test and resides in an area endemic for HIV.

Screening for hepatitis viruses at mental health and substance abuse agencies appears to be spotty, as is screening for most medical problems. Mental health agencies that have established medical services on-site (e.g., inpatient units or shelters with co-located primary care clinics) may screen automatically for HCV and sometimes hepatitis B virus in routine laboratory examinations. In the vast majority of mental health agencies lacking on-site medical services, providers know about HCV infection only if patients self-report having been diagnosed or if they are in such advanced stages as to manifest signs of liver failure (e.g., spider angiomata, jaundice, ascites).

The initial diagnosis of HIV infection may occur when a patient first becomes infected, in advanced AIDS, or at any time in between. Shock and disbelief may be followed by depression, anxiety, and fear in adjusting to having contracted a serious and still potentially deadly illness. In many nonindustrialized countries AIDS remains a rapidly terminal condition. Untreated depression and hopelessness may be associated with continuing risk behavior, even suicidal ideation (Liberman et al. 1986). Like serious mental illness, HIV and AIDS can be highly stigmatizing, possibly resulting in rejection, abandonment, and further social isolation. If a worsening of psychiatric symptoms follows the initial HIV diagnosis, the most effective intervention is individual counseling and supportive therapy geared to both the current mental status of the patient and his or her knowledge and understanding of HIV infection (Broder et al. 1994).

Legal regulations or guidelines for confidentiality and the disclosure of HIV- or AIDS-related information are in place in many countries and can set the stage for upholding humane and responsible individual and public health standards. Contact notification by physicians may not be required, but legal statutes may allow doctors or public health officers to notify the contact themselves if they determine that a patient will not inform a contact who is at significant risk. Laws that are applicable to the locality should be consulted in making decisions that involve confidentiality and contact notification.

Testing for HCV can occur at any point and does not require a special consent. Nonetheless, it remains important to explain the test result to patients found to be HCV positive and to refer such patients for further evaluation and, as appropriate, hepatitis A and B virus immunization.

For HIV-infected psychiatric patients who are asymptomatic, supportive groups may encourage behavioral change and promote ways to preserve physical health in the community and within the psychiatric setting. This kind of group intervention can prevent worsening of psychiatric symptoms and provide a sense of community that can decrease social isolation, reinforce safer peer norms, and encourage altruism, which appeals to ego strengths and gives patients a sense of worth and accomplishment.

Although most outpatient agencies in New York City, an early epicenter, distribute HIV educational material, half or fewer of these service settings provide risk reduction interventions, conduct risk assessments, offer pre- and posttest counseling, or hold support groups for HIV-positive patients. The reason for this may be unmet needs for training, reported by 84% of agencies that serve between 1 and 10 persons with HIV infection annually and have staff members already trained in providing at least one HIV-related service. Services may be directed at patients on the basis of their suspected or presumed risks rather than on the basis of a thorough risk assessment (McKinnon et al. 1999, 2001). These findings are echoed in other United States regions (e.g., Brunette et al. 2000) and may suggest how to improve service delivery systems in other AIDS-endemic areas where resources allow for comprehensive care.

Clinicians may be in the best position to help their patients access HIV testing, treatment, and prevention opportunities. They can employ many strategies to help their patients determine their risk of acquiring or transmitting the AIDS virus; to prevent new infections, to promote healthier behaviors; and to reduce the impact of HIV-related illness on this vulnerable population. They also are uniquely qualified to help their patients manage the many medications required to maintain their psychiatric and physical health.

Rational Psychopharmacology for People With HIV/ HCV and Schizophrenia

HIV-related psychopharmacological interventions for people with preexisting schizophrenia follow similar guidelines for patients with new-onset psychosis associated with HIV infection. In advanced HIV infection, traditional neuroleptic agents have been found to produce modest but significant reductions in psychotic symptoms but have been eschewed for newer, atypical antipsychotics for the primary reason that such patients are very sensitive to extrapyramidal side effects due to viral involvement of the basal ganglia (American Psychiatric Association 2000; Fernandez and Levy 1993; Sewell et al. 1994). With progression of HIV, people with preexisting psychiatric conditions may thus develop new or increased side effects on medications that they were previously able to tolerate (Horwath 1996).

A large number of medications are prescribed to people with HIV infection, including antibacterial, antifungal, antineoplastic, antiretroviral, and other antiviral agents (Horwath 1996), particularly in later stages of HIV disease, when numerous present or potential complications require active treatment or prophylaxis. Any attempt to diagnose drug-induced neuropsychiatric syndromes requires an appreciation of both the therapeutic use and potential side effects of these medications. Some of these are described in the Practice Guideline for the Treatment of Patients With HIV/AIDS of the American Psychiatric Association (2000; access at www.psych.org), but new antiretroviral agents are being developed at a rapid pace, and existing medications to treat HIV-related infections and neoplasms are too numerous to describe fully. Neuropsychiatric side effects of antiretrovirals have been reported most commonly with efavirenz (Sustiva) and occasionally with nevirapine (Viramune). There are many in vitro predictions of drug-drug interactions (which can be found in hand-held databases, those available through hospital pharmacies, and those online at a variety of Web sites), but experienced prescribers generally find they can use the full range of psychotropic medications if they start with low doses and slowly increase the medication. Overlapping toxicities between different medications must also be taken into consideration. It is important to be aware that advanced HIV infection is associated with greater sensitivity to both the therapeutic effects and side effects of psychotropic medications, which is another reason why it is best to start with the lowest possible doses and increase medications slowly. Drug levels, if available, should be monitored closely, especially when patients are on complex medication regimens. Recreational drugs also can affect medication levels; for dually diagnosed patients on methadone, doses of methadone often need to be adjusted, usually upward but occasionally downward depending on the antiretroviral regimen (i.e., delavirdine, nevirapine).

Most psychiatric medications are metabolized by the liver and therefore may require more careful monitoring in those chronically infected with hepatitis C. In particular, for those who manifest clinical or laboratory signs of liver failure, medication metabolism can be dangerously reduced to the point where patients may accumulate toxic levels of drugs they normally can take.

In general, it is relatively safe to use most of the psychiatric medications both with HIV and HCV treatments. In the presence of HCV illness,

periodic liver function tests are the standard of care. Because some psychotropics may elevate liver enzymes (e.g., valproic acid, carbamazepine,
nefazodone), it is important to check these at baseline, early after initiation
of therapy (2–4 weeks), and every 2–3 months thereafter. Nevertheless,
data from a large retrospective study in Seattle, Washington, found that
among 94 HCV seropositive patients treated with valproic acid, 81.9%
showed minimal or no evidence of serum transaminase elevations (Barnes
et al. 2001). Yet combined toxicities are important to consider, particularly
during treatment with medications that can have an impact on bone marrow
activity (e.g., clozapine, carbamazepine, zidovudine, interferon, ribavirin) or
may cause other additive side effects. Initiating interferon treatment
should involve follow-up by a psychiatrist, both to evaluate the patient
with schizophrenia as a candidate for long-term interferon on the basis of
compliance with psychiatric therapy, and to monitor for psychiatric symptom exacerbation.

Psychiatric patients, like medical patients, often are nonadherent to
their medication regimen, which they may perceive as one of the few aspects of their lives they can control. It is important to time the beginning
of an antiretroviral regimen with a commitment to the treatment and to
help patients see that following an HIV or HCV medication regimen can
be part of gaining control. Working with a patient to promote adherence
to psychotropic medications will be the best predictor of whether the patient can follow an HIV/HCV medication regimen. The clinician and infectious disease specialist must communicate about the patient's need for
and readiness to begin antiretrovirals, select in concert with the patient
regimens that avoid drug–drug interactions, keep the number and doses
of pills the patient has to take to the minimum necessary, and coordinate
his or her treatment plans.

Conclusion

Understanding the HIV and HCV epidemics and their underpinnings
among people with severe mental illness can help clinicians to recognize
when their patients with schizophrenia are at risk for acquiring or transmitting these viruses and to intervene appropriately and effectively with preventive, counseling and testing, medical, and supportive services. It is critical for
clinicians to receive training to enhance their knowledge and skills in these
areas, to ask comfortably and nonjudgmentally about their patients' risks
rather than waiting until patients are ill to learn about risk behaviors, and
continually to access up-to-date information and technical assistance about
how to prevent and treat these infections among their patients.

References

Acuda SW, Sebit MB: Serostatus surveillance testing of HIV-I infection among Zimbabwean psychiatric inpatients in Zimbabwe. Cent Afr J Med 42:254–257, 1996

American Psychiatric Association: Practice Guideline for the Treatment of Patients with HIV/AIDS. Am J Psychiatry 157 (suppl):1–62, 2000

Ayuso-Mateos JL, Montanes F, Lastra I, et al: HIV infection in psychiatric patients: an unlinked anonymous study. Br J Psychiatry 170:181–185, 1997

Barnes R, Felker B, Sloan K, et al: Safety of valproic acid treatment in patients with hepatitis C. Poster presented at the 40th annual meeting of the American College of Neuropsychopharmacology, Waikoloa, HI, December 9, 2001

Barre-Sinoussi F, Chermann JC, Rey F, et al: Isolation of a T-lymphotropic retrovirus from a patient at risk for acquired immunodeficiency syndrome. Science 220:868–871, 1983

Broder S, Merigan TC, Bolognesi D (eds): Textbook of AIDS Medicine. Baltimore, MD, Williams & Wilkins, 1994

Brunette MF, Mercer CC, Carlson CL, et al: HIV-related services for persons with severe mental illness: policy and practice in New Hampshire community mental health. J Behav Health Serv Res 27:347–353, 2000

Carey MP, Carey KB, Kalichman SC: Risk for human immunodeficiency virus (HIV) infection among persons with severe mental illnesses. Clin Psychol Rev 17:271–291, 1997

Carmen E, Brady SM: AIDS risk and prevention for the chronic mentally ill. Hosp Community Psychiatry 41:652–657, 1990

Chuang HT, Atkinson M: AIDS knowledge and high-risk behaviour in the chronic mentally ill. Can J Psychiatry 41:269–272, 1996

Cividini A, Pistorio A, Regazzetti A, et al: Hepatitis C virus infection among institutionalized psychiatric patients: a regression analysis of indicators of risk. J Hepatol 27:455–463, 1997

Community Research Initiative on AIDS: HIV/hepatitis C co-infection: confronting twin epidemics. http://www.CRIANY.org, accessed January 2000

Corbitt G, Crosdale E, Bailey A: Protracted sero-conversion in haemophiliacs in whom infection is confirmed by p24 antigen detection and/or positive HIV PCR, in Abstracts, 7th International Conference on AIDS, Florence, Italy, 1991, p 387

Cournos F, McKinnon K: HIV seroprevalence among people with severe mental illness in the United States: a critical review. Clin Psychol Rev 17:259–269, 1997

Cournos F, Guido JR, Coomaraswamy S, et al: Sexual activity and risk of HIV infection among patients with schizophrenia. Am J Psychiatry 151:228–232, 1993

Fernandez F, Levy JK: The use of molindone in the treatment of psychotic and delirious patients infected with the human immunodeficiency virus: case reports. Gen Hosp Psychiatry 15:31–35, 1993

Gallo RC, Salahuddin SZ, Popovic M, et al: Frequent detection and isolation of cy-topathic retroviruses (HTLV-III) from patients with AIDS and at risk for AIDS. Science 224:500–503, 1984

Goodman LA, Fallot RD: HIV risk-behavior in poor urban women with serious mental disorders: association with childhood physical and sexual abuse. Am J Orthopsychiatry 68:73–83, 1998

Hanson M, Kramer TH, Gross W, et al: AIDS awareness and risk behaviors among dually disordered adults. AIDS Educ Prev 4:41–51, 1992

Hardy AM: National health interview survey data on adult knowledge about AIDS in the United States. Public Health Rep 105:629–634, 1990

Herbert B: Woman battering and HIV infection, in Abstracts (TP500), HIV Infec-tion in Women: Setting a New Agenda. Washington, DC, Philadelphia Sci-ences Group, 1995

Horwath E: Psychiatric and neuropsychiatric manifestations, in AIDS and People With Severe Mental Illness: A Handbook for Mental Health Professionals. Edited by Cournos F, Bakalar N. New Haven, CT, Yale University Press, 1996, pp 57–73

Horwath E, Cournos F, McKinnon K, et al: Illicit-drug injection among psychiatric patients without a primary substance use disorder. Psychiatr Serv 47:181–185, 1996

Kalichman SC, Kelly JA, Johnson JR, et al: Factors associated with risk for HIV in-fection among chronic mentally ill adults. Am J Psychiatry 151:221–227, 1994

Katz RC, Watts C, Santman J: AIDS knowledge and high risk behaviors in the chronic mentally ill. Community Ment Health J 30:395–402, 1994

Keet IP, Krol A, Koot M, et al: Predictors of rapid progression to AIDS in HIV-1 seroconverters. AIDS 7:51–57, 1993

Kelly JA: HIV risk reduction interventions for persons with severe mental illness. Clin Psychol Rev 17:293–309, 1997

Kelly JA, Murphy DA, Bahr GR, et al: AIDS/HIV risk behavior among the chronic mentally ill. Am J Psychiatry 149:886–889, 1992

Levy J: Pathogenesis of human immunodeficiency virus infection. Microbiol Rev 57:183–189, 1993

Liberman RP, Mueser KT, Wallace CJ, et al: Training skills in the psychiatrically disabled: learning coping and competence. Schizophr Bull 12:631–647, 1986

Lifson AR, Buchbinder SP, Sheppard HW, et al: Long-term human immunodefi-ciency virus infection in asymptomatic homosexual and bisexual men with normal CD4+ lymphocyte counts: immunologic and virologic characteristics. J Infect Dis 163:959–965, 1991

Masliah G, Achim CL, DeTeresa R, et al: The patterns of neurodegeneration in HIV encephalitis. Journal of NeuroAIDS 1:161–173, 1996

McDaniel JS, Purcell DW, Farber EW: Severe mental illness and HIV-related medical and neuropsychiatric sequelae. Clin Psychol Rev 17:311–325, 1997

McDermott BE, Sautter FJ, Winstead DK, et al: Diagnosis, health beliefs, and risk of HIV infection in psychiatric patients. Hosp Community Psychiatry 45:580–585, 1994

McKinnon K, Cournos F: HIV infection linked to substance use among hospitalized patients with severe mental illness. Psychiatr Serv 49:1269, 1998

McKinnon K, Cournos F, Sugden R, et al: The relative contributions of psychiatric symptoms and AIDS knowledge to HIV risk behaviors among people with severe mental illness. J Clin Psychiatry 57:506–513, 1996

McKinnon K, Cournos F, Herman R, et al: AIDS-related services and training in outpatient mental health care agencies in New York. Psychiatr Serv 50:1225–1228, 1999

McKinnon K, Wainberg ML, Cournos F: HIV/AIDS preparedness in mental health care agencies with high and low substance use disorder caseloads. J Subst Abuse 13:127–135, 2001

Mellors JW, Rinaldo CR Jr, Gupta P, et al: Prognosis in HIV-1 infection predicted by the quantity of virus in plasma. Science 272:1167–1170, 1996

Menon AS, Pomerantz S: Substance use during sex and unsafe sexual behaviors among acute psychiatric inpatients. Psychiatr Serv 48:1070–1072, 1997

Meyer JM: Prevalence of hepatitis A, hepatitis B and HIV among hepatitis C seropositive state hospital patients: results from Oregon State Hospital. J Clin Psychiatry (in press)

Mulder RT, Ang M, Chapman B, et al: Interferon treatment is not associated with a worsening of psychiatric symptoms in patients with hepatitis C. J Gastroenterol Hepatol 15: 300–303, 2000

National Digestive Diseases Information Clearinghouse: Chronic hepatitis C: current disease management. Available at: http://www.niddk.nih.gov/health/digest/pubs/chrnhepc. Accessed February 17, 2003

National Institutes of Health Consensus Development Conference Panel: Management of hepatitis C. Hepatology 26:2S–10S, 1997

O'Brien WA: Genetic and biologic basis of HIV-1 neurotropism, in HIV, AIDS and the Brain. Edited by Price RW, Perry SW. New York, Raven, 1994, pp 47–70

O'Brien WA, Hartigan PM, Martin D, et al: Changes in plasma HIV-1 RNA and CD4 + lymphocyte counts and the risk of progression to AIDS. N Engl J Med 334:426–431, 1996

Oliveira SB: Avaliação do comportamento sexual, conhecimentos e atitudes sobre AIDS, dos pacientes internados no instituto de psiquiatria da UFRJ, in O Campo da Atenção Psicossocial. Edited by Venâncio AT, Leal EM, Delgado PG. Rio de Janeiro, Te Corá, 1997, pp 343–351

Oquendo M, Tricarico P: Pre- and post-HIV test counseling, in AIDS and People With Severe Mental Illness: A Handbook for Mental Health Professionals. Edited by Cournos F, Bakalar N. New Haven, CT, Yale University Press, 1996, pp 97–112

Otto-Salaj LL, Heckman TG, Stevenson LY, et al: Patterns, predictors and gender differences in HIV risk among severely mentally ill men and women. Community Ment Health J 34:175–190, 1998

Otto-Salaj LL, Kelly JA, Stevenson LY, et al: Outcomes of a randomized small-group HIV prevention intervention trial for people with serious mental illness. Community Ment Health J 37:123–144, 2001

Resnick L, Berger JR, Shapshak P, et al: Early penetration of the blood brain barrier by HTLV-III/LAV. Neurology 38:9–15, 1988

Rosenberg SD, Goodman LA, Osher FC, et al: Prevalence of HIV, hepatitis B, and hepatitis C in people with severe mental illness. Am J Public Health 91:31–37, 2001

Sewell DD, Jeste DV, McAdams LA, et al: Neuroleptic treatment of HIV-associated psychosis. Neuropsychopharmacology 10:223–229, 1994

Staprans SI, Feinberg MB: Natural history and immunopathogenesis of HIV-1 disease, in The Medical Management of AIDS, 5th Edition. Edited by Sande MA, Volberding PA. Philadelphia, PA, WB Saunders, 1997, pp 29–56

Susser E, Miller M, Valencia E, et al: Injection drug use and risk of HIV transmission among homeless men with mental illness. Am J Psychiatry 153:794–798, 1996

Varmus H: Retroviruses. Science 240:1427–1435, 1988

Vento S, Garofano T, Renzini C, et al: Fulminant hepatitis associated with hepatitis A virus superinfection in patients with chronic hepatitis C. N Engl J Med 338:286–290, 1998

Wainberg ML, Forstein M, Berkman A, et al: Essential medical facts for mental health practitioners, in What Mental Health Practitioners Need to Know about HIV and AIDS. Edited by Cournos F, Forstein M. San Francisco, CA, Jossey-Bass, 2000, pp 3–15

Warner GC: Molecular insights into HIV-1 infection, in The Medical Management of AIDS, 5th Edition. Edited by Sande MA, Volberding PA. Philadelphia, PA, WB Saunders, 1997, pp 17–28

Chapter 8

Medical Health in Aging Persons With Schizophrenia

Raymelle Schoos, M.D.
Carl I. Cohen, M.D.

Introduction

A potential health crisis is emerging in mental health care. Approximately 2% of the population over age 54—about 1 million persons—suffer from chronic mental illness other than dementia, the majority of them diagnosed with schizophrenia (Cohen et al. 2000). Over the next 30 years this number will double as postwar baby-boomers reach old age; these individuals will also be at increased risk for physical illness as they age. More than four-fifths of the general older population are affected by one or more chronic medical conditions (Kovar 2001), and disease combinations can act synergistically to produce a much higher level of functional disability

This work was supported in part by grant no. SO6 GM54650 from the National Institute of General Medical Sciences.

than that associated with either disease alone (Verbrugge et al. 1991). Thus, physical disease co-occurring with schizophrenia may have a greater impact on adaptive functioning than it would in persons without mental disease. Unlike previous generations of older schizophrenic persons, who spent much of their later years in mental institutions, approximately 85% of older schizophrenic persons now live in the community, in settings other than nursing homes or hospitals (Cohen et al. 2000). A critical issue for the new generation of older schizophrenic persons is whether they will be able to negotiate health and social service systems that may be ill prepared to deal with them.

The aim of this chapter is to provide an overview of medical health issues of aging schizophrenic persons. We first focus on the epidemiology of physical disorders, both general physical health and specific medical disorders. Next we examine treatment issues, including medication-related issues, barriers to health care, and concerns about competency.

Background

Few papers have specifically addressed issues of health among aging individuals with schizophrenia, with a recent review by Cohen et al. (2000) finding only 1% of the literature on schizophrenia devoted to issues of aging. Research in this area has been limited by the fact that the majority of schizophrenia studies cover a wide age range, with the predominant focus on younger patients. Comparisons between studies are also hampered by the differences in types of patients (inpatient versus outpatient, Veterans Affairs [VA] hospitals), use of disease prevalence rather than incidence in populations, and diverse geographical locations for the study populations. Despite these limitations, we have tried in this chapter, wherever possible, to make comparisons between older schizophrenic persons and their age peers in the general population or with other psychiatric populations, and to make comparisons between older and younger schizophrenic persons. To expand our data sources, we have also extrapolated from studies of schizophrenic persons in general by using mean values and standard deviations and by incorporating any findings in which there is a breakdown by age.

General Physical Health

It is generally believed that schizophrenic persons have worse health than their age peers in the general population, and that their conditions often go undiagnosed and untreated (Dixon et al. 1999). For example, increased rates of comorbid physical illness in schizophrenic patients have been reported to occur primarily in the categories of non–insulin-dependent diabetes mellitus (NIDDM), cardiovascular disease, infectious diseases, respiratory disease, some forms of cancer, and a variety of other illnesses (Dixon et al. 1999). It has also been suggested that persons with schizophrenia may be subject to more severe forms of disorders (Jeste et al. 1996), which may be exacerbated by the side effects of antipsychotic medications (e.g., anticholinergic, cardiovascular, or metabolic effects) and by psychotic illness itself, with significant correlations found between positive symptoms and the number of medical conditions (Dixon et al. 1999; Jeste et al. 1996).

Because data suggest that the diagnosis of schizophrenia across all age ranges confers greater risk for physical illness, it might be assumed that older persons with schizophrenia are more medically ill than age-matched peers. Moreover, it is conceivable that age may interact with schizophrenia so that older schizophrenic persons might be disproportionately more ill relative to their age peers than younger schizophrenic persons.

Nevertheless, researchers in San Diego (Jeste et al. 1996; Lacro and Jeste 1994) found that middle-aged and older schizophrenic persons had fewer medical illnesses (mean = 1.0) than persons with Alzheimer's disease (mean = 1.4) and major depression (mean = 2.4), with a comparable severity index on the Cumulative Illness Rating Scale for Geriatrics (CIRS-G) compared with an older normal comparison group. Similarly, a study in New York City of 117 schizophrenic persons age 55 and over, with a mean age of 63 years (C.I. Cohen, unpublished data), found that 33% of the schizophrenia sample and 48% of the community sample reported 2 or more physical disorders; the mean number of disorders was 1.35 and 1.66 for the schizophrenia and community groups, respectively. In the latter studies, the annual rate of hospitalization was comparable between the groups (21% community group, 22% schizophrenia group), although more than half the hospitalizations among the schizophrenia group had been for psychiatric reasons, whereas among the community sample only about 1 in 20 hospitalizations had been psychiatric in nature. However, a confounding factor in both of these investigations was that the normal comparison groups were older—12 years and 6 years in the San Diego and New York City studies, respectively. Interestingly, the San Diego study found a significant correlation between physical symptom severity and positive symptoms of schizophrenia, depression, and overall psychopathology, whereas the New York study did not find any significant correlations.

The studies in New York and San Diego do not suggest that older schizophrenic outpatients have more physical disorders or that their disorders are necessarily more severe than those of their age peers from comparable backgrounds, although results of the latter study were equivocal due to age differences between comparison groups. One possible explanation for these findings is that persons in the schizophrenia samples were all involved to some extent in clinical programs, most of which encouraged or provided physical examinations. Moreover, because aspects of psychopathology tend to diminish with age, older persons may be more apt to attend to medical problems and be better received by other health professionals. The San Diego researchers interpreted the significant correlation between positive symptoms and physical health as reflecting the fact that physical symptoms may seem less important or be overlooked in the presence of florid psychosis and, conversely, are more apt to be addressed when the patient is less symptomatic. A "survivor effect" may be another plausible explanation for the lack of differences between the older schizophrenic and community persons. That is, because the mortality rate for schizophrenic persons substantially exceeds that of the general population throughout their lifetime, those who are oldest are presumably the heartiest, both physically and emotionally.

Specific Medical Disorders

Diabetes

The association between diabetes and schizophrenia is discussed at length in Chapter 6 of this volume. Nonetheless, it bears noting that despite the fact that diabetes increases with age and affects about 20% of the geriatric population (Marsh 1997), the prevalence rate of diabetes among schizophrenia patients versus persons without psychiatric illness seems to be consistently higher only in younger and middle-aged groups, with differences in the geriatric population less apparent. Jeste et al. (1996) found no significant difference in the prevalence of diabetes when comparing a group of middle-aged and elderly schizophrenic patients with individuals with other psychiatric disorders. Similar results were found in a study of older schizophrenic persons in New York City, in which self-reported rates of diabetes were nearly identical between schizophrenic persons (20%) and the comparison community group (19%) (C.I. Cohen, unpublished data). Two studies (Mukherjee 1995) of VA inpatients and outpatients have confirmed the increasing prevalence of diabetes among schizophrenic persons as they age, with rates of 0% and 1.6% among those under 40, and 25% and 50% in those 70 years and above, for inpatients and outpatients, respectively. In another study, conducted in Italy, Mukherjee et al. (1996) studied a sample of 95 schizophrenic patients and found that the prevalence of diabetes increased from 0% in those younger than 50 years to 12.9% in those age 50–59 years, 18.9% in those age 60–69 years, and 16.7% in the 70–74 age group.

Although antipsychotic medication, particularly the atypical agents olanzapine and clozapine, may have an impact on glucose tolerance, the Patient Outcomes Research Team (PORT) study concluded that the risk of developing diabetes in schizophrenic patients exceeded the general population's risk even before the widespread use of the newer agents (Dixon et al. 2000). Similarly, Mukherjee et al. (1996) observed, "More critically it bears emphasizing that high rates of insulin resistance and impaired glucose tolerance had been noted in schizophrenia patients before the introduction of neuroleptics" (p. 71).

With respect to treatment, the PORT study, based on data from 719 schizophrenic outpatients (mean age 43 years and approximately 17% above age 55), found that 86% of schizophrenia patients who reported having diabetes mellitus said they were receiving treatment for it (Dixon et al. 1999). This is consistent with data from the study of older schizophrenic persons in New York City that was cited earlier, in which 85% of persons with diabetes reported receiving treatment for this disorder.

Cardiovascular Disease

Cardiovascular diseases are among the most common disorders found among schizophrenic persons. Cardiovascular disease is reported to occur more frequently and to be responsible for increased mortality rates in schizophrenic individuals versus those in the general population (Dixon et al. 1999; Tsuang et al. 1983). The Oxford Record Linkage Study (ORLS), which used data derived from hospital activity analyses and mental health inquiry systems, included 2,314 persons with schizophrenia across all age groups, of whom one-third were age 55 or older. For these patients there was a significant increase in relative risk for atherosclerotic heart disease, but not for other forms of cardiac, hypertensive, or other circulatory diseases (Baldwin 1979).

The limited data on older schizophrenic samples have been more mixed than the findings for schizophrenia in general. Sajatovic et al. (1996) studied 49 schizophrenic patients at the Cleveland Veterans Affairs Medical Center ranging in age from 65 to 85 with a mean age of 72 years (96% were male). They reported that the most frequent reasons for medical hospitalization in their schizophrenic patients were cardiovascular or pulmonary disease, although there was no comparison with nonpsychiatric patients. Sheline (1990) reported that cardiovascular disease was the most prevalent physical illness seen in a sample of geriatric psychiatric inpatients consisting of 95 patients (57 women and 38 men) between the ages of 60 and 85. Although schizophrenics accounted for 20% of the study population, the data for the study were not further broken down to examine medical diagnoses specific to those with schizophrenia. Lacro and Jeste (1994) compared elderly schizophrenic patients with other elderly psychiatric patients and found that the schizophrenic patients had the lowest prevalence of hypertension, coronary artery disease, and congestive heart failure. Finally, in the New York City study of older schizophrenic outpatients cited previously, self-reported rates of heart conditions were lower than those in a community comparison group (20% vs. 26%), and hypertension was dramatically lower than in the community group (29% vs. 57%).

Respiratory Disorders

Until 50 years ago, respiratory diseases such as pneumonia and tuberculosis accounted for much of the excessive mortality rates among institutionalized schizophrenic patients (Alstrom 1942; Baldwin 1979; Odegaard 1951). It should be pointed out that these findings were not specific to schizophrenic patients, but rather were observed in institutionalized psychiatric patients as a whole. Recent studies, however, continue to point to disproportionately high rates of respiratory morbidity and mortality in schizophrenic populations, although the usual proviso about lack of data among older schizophrenic persons obtains here as well.

Respiratory disease was found to be one of the most common causes of medical hospitalization (18%, compared with 22% for cardiovascular disease) in the 10-year study by Sajatovic et al. (1996) of hospital utilization by elderly veterans with bipolar disorder ($n=23$) and schizophrenia ($n=49$). Hussar (1966) examined the autopsy reports of 1,275 chronic white male schizophrenic patients with a mean age at the time of death of 63 years, collected from 29 VA hospitals, and found an increased number of deaths due to pneumonia versus the age-matched rate of the general population. Weiner and Marvit (1977) found increased morbidity from respiratory disease in their middle-aged schizophrenia population, and Dynes (1969) and Saku et al. (1995) found respiratory disease to be a leading cause of death in their schizophrenic population of all ages.

Immune Function

Hypotheses about the link between immune dysfunction and schizophrenia date back to the early twentiethth century, and in the 1960s an autoimmune-mediated process was implicated in the etiology of schizophrenia (Rappaport and Delrahim 2001). Paradoxically, however, studies of specific immunological disorders have generally supported lower prevalence rates among schizophrenic populations. For example, Ehrentheil (1957) and Lipper and Werman (1977) have noted a decreased incidence of asthma, hay fever, and other allergic reactions in schizophrenic patients. Other studies, such as Sabbath and Luce (1952), showed an alternating pattern of coexisting psychosis and allergies.

The strongest evidence for a negative association between schizophrenia and a disease exists for rheumatoid arthritis (RA). Nissen and Spencer (1936) may have been the first to point out that RA and schizophrenia do not appear to exist together. Eaton et al. (1992) reviewed 14 epidemiological studies conducted between 1934 and 1985 and concluded that there was ample evidence to support the negative association between these two disorders. Baldwin (1979), Tsuang et al. (1983), and Allebeck (1989) are further examples of studies finding a low relative risk between the two disorders. Underdiagnosis has been proposed as one explanation for the negative association observed between schizophrenia and RA (Mors et al. 1999).

Cancer

Increased and decreased prevalence rates for different types of cancer among schizophrenic populations have been reported in the literature. Comparisons are made more difficult because some studies focus on death rates and others focus on disease rates. In general, compared with the overall population, there seems to be a pattern of lower rates of lung cancer and higher rates of digestive and breast cancers among schizophrenic populations (Schoos and Cohen 2003). The apparent lower prevalence of lung cancer in schizophrenia patients is surprising in light of the high prevalence of smoking in this population (Jeste et al. 1996); however, a more recent British study of 370 schizophrenic patients ages 16–66 (Brown et al. 2000) found mortality rates for lung cancer in schizophrenic persons to be twice the expected values. The fact that the majority of these patients were also heavy smokers raises the likelihood that cigarette smoking may indeed account for the higher mortality rate.

Looking at age-specific trends, Mortensen and Juel (1993) concluded that there is no significant increase in cancer mortality in any age group of schizophrenic persons, but there is a trend toward decreased mortality in older patients. Based on a schizophrenic study population consisting of 555 females (65% 60 years of age or older) and 389 males (81% 60 years or older), Malzberg (1950) found increased cancer mortality in young patients with mental illness but significantly decreased rates in elderly patients, with lower rates among males. Baldwin (1979) reported that long-term hospitalized elderly patients had significant reductions in lung cancer, gastrointestinal cancer, and prostate/bladder cancer. There appears to be excess cancer mortality in mental patients as a whole when hospital stays are short, whereas cancer mortality rates are diminished versus the general population when hospital stays are long, especially among those age 65 or older (Baldwin 1979; Fox and Howell 1974). However, although these studies included schizophrenia patients, they were not specific to schizophrenia. Baldwin (1979) posits two possible explanations for the increase in mortality rates among short-stay patients, including greater age or reasons for the admission (i.e., selective processes). Lower cancer mortality rates among longer-stay older persons has led some authors to propose that the environment of the hospital, rather than schizophrenia per se, could be a factor in protecting schizophrenic elderly persons from some cancers (Tsuang et al. 1983).

Controversial data exist with respect to neuroleptic use and cancer morbidity/mortality. Mortensen (1986) proposed that phenothiazine treatment may be an environmental factor that protects against malignant neoplasia. High-dose neuroleptics have been associated with reduced incidence of bladder and prostate cancer, and non-phenothiazine neuroleptics with a decrease in lung and breast cancer (Mortensen 1989, 1992; Mortensen and Juel 1990). However, on the opposite side, Ettigi et al. (1973) observed that breast cancer may be more common with phenothiazine treatment. Goode et al. (1981) suggested that neuroleptics may potentially cause the increased incidence of breast cancer by elevating the prolactin level, although their study in a large psychiatric hospital over a decade noted that breast cancer rates were not higher among these psychiatric patients despite their use of antipsychotic drugs.

Hyponatremia

Older persons, in general, are at greater risk for developing hyponatremia, with data suggesting that older persons with schizophrenia have an even greater susceptibility. A study by de Leon et al. (1994) suggested that up to 20% of chronically institutionalized schizophrenic patients may suffer from polydipsia, and Jos et al. (1986) found that polydipsia was seen most frequently in white male schizophrenic inpatients.

It has been theorized that persons with schizophrenia may have increased antidiuretic hormone (ADH) release and abnormal osmotic regulation, or that the effects of antipsychotic medications on ADH release result in hyponatremia. One study noted that 70% of hyponatremic schizophrenic patients were taking anticholinergic drugs versus 8% of the normonatremic schizophrenic patients, leading to the conclusion that dryness of mucous membranes induces thirst and increased water consumption. Given that most schizophrenic patients are heavy smokers, the stimulating effects of nicotine on ADH release may also play a role.

Mortality Rates

With respect to general mortality rates, most studies agree that older schizophrenic patients have lower-than-expected mortality in relation to other older psychiatric patients, but still have increased mortality in comparison with the general population. Possible explanations for this include a different sort of lifestyle (environment) for schizophrenic patients, a possible protective mechanism of neuroleptics on cardiovascular function, and the fact that elderly schizophrenic patients are survivors in that they have made it through a weeding-out process in which other physically ill schizophrenic patients have died. The lower mortality in older schizophrenic persons is observed for nearly all causes, the exceptions being heart disease and cancer (Wood et al. 1985).

Subjective Health Status

Self-rated health status is an important measure of subjective well-being. Although it tends to correlate with more objective measures of health, it is based on personal perception and judgment. These may be influenced by health problems in the past, the level of health of other persons in the subject's social sphere, and the subject's aspirations for the future. Thus, certain persons may underestimate the severity of their illnesses and postpone seeking treatment.

There have been only a few studies examining this issue in aging schizophrenic populations. One study by Krach (1993) used the Older Americans Resources Survey to obtain information from 20 older schizophrenic patients, with a mean age of 61 years, on physical health. Ratings of excellent/good and fair/poor physical health were reported by 60% and 40% of the sample, respectively. Mental health ratings were similar, with 70% and 30% reporting excellent/good and fair/poor mental health, respectively. Based on the level of physical disorders and reports of impairment in activities of daily living (ADL) (e.g., 35% had moderate or severe ADL impairment),

Krach concluded that these patients overrated their physical health status and underreported medical symptoms, although the author provided no objective measures of physical health. Indeed, in contradistinction to Krach's conclusions, the authors of the PORT study (Dixon et al. 1999) maintained that "persons with schizophrenia have the capacity for reasonable appraisal of their medical conditions that can be a useful tool to promote positive health behaviors" (p. 502). This conclusion was based on the finding of a significant association between the number of medical conditions and self-rated health. In the PORT survey, lower educational level and number of comorbid medical disorders were the only variables associated with poorer self-rated physical health. Other variables, such as gender, race, age, comorbid alcohol or drug disorder, geographic location, or patient setting, were not associated with self-health ratings, although there was a trend for older subjects to perceive their health as better.

The study of older schizophrenic persons in New York City cited previously found that despite equal or lower prevalence rates of physical disorders among schizophrenic persons compared with older community persons, self-reported health differed between the two aging samples (C.I. Cohen, unpublished data). When the entire schizophrenic sample was examined, the percentage reporting excellent/good health was 38%, compared with 54% of community persons. In a multivariate analysis, only activity limitations and depression were significant predictors of negative self-health ratings among older schizophrenic persons. Compared with the general older community sample, older schizophrenic persons had higher scores on the scales for depression (7.5 vs. 5.5) and activity limitations (6.0 vs. 5.0), although it is worth noting that scores on the activity scale can be affected by limitations due to mental as well as physical causes. Thus, the results of the multivariate analysis indicate that self-health ratings may primarily reflect psychological rather than physical factors. Moreover, it suggests that older schizophrenic persons do not overestimate their physical well-being versus their age peers in the community, and, if anything, they may underrate their own physical well-being.

Treatment Issues

Pharmacokinetic and Pharmacodynamic Factors

Because older schizophrenic persons are usually receiving antipsychotic medications, the addition of drugs for physical disorders or other psychotropic drugs requires a sophisticated understanding of the potential risks for adverse effects. Here we briefly summarize some basic concepts of pharmacokinetics and pharmacodynamics as they affect older persons in general.

Pharmacokinetics, or how a drug moves through the body, becomes increasingly important with advancing age. Age affects the absorption, distribution, metabolism, and elimination of medications to varying degrees (Jacobson et al. 2002). Absorption may be affected by physiological changes associated with aging, including decreased gastric acidity, a decline in small bowel surface area, and diminished blood flow to the small bowel. However, no clinically significant decreases in drug absorption attributable to aging have been reported. Nonetheless, use of antacids, fiber supplements, or anticholinergic agents may slow absorption and delay the onset of medication action.

Distribution of drugs to peripheral sites is substantially affected by aging, as adipose tissue increases and lean body mass decreases. Thus, there is a larger volume of distribution for fat-soluble drugs, which includes nearly all psychotropic medications. There are several consequences to this age-related change: the half-life of lipophilic drugs increases, leading to the accumulation of drugs taken chronically and thus to greater potential for toxicity; increased uptake in the peripheral sites (e.g., fat tissues) may result in less drug reaching the brain and in a potentially shorter duration of drug action after a single dose than is seen in younger persons. Conversely, total body water decreases with age so that the volume of distribution of water-soluble drugs decreases, more of the drug is present in the circulation, and proportionately more reaches the brain. Thus, water-soluble drugs such as ethanol and lithium may have increased effects in older persons. Elderly persons also have a diminished lean body mass, so drugs such as digoxin that bind to muscle may show increased concentrations at any given strength. Finally, the concentration of plasma proteins such as albumin tends to decrease in older persons, and this decline may be exacerbated by physical illness and poor nutrition. For protein-bound drugs, lower albumin concentrations affect the free fraction (percent bound vs. unbound) but do not affect the measured total drug concentration. The principal concern is that laboratory measurement of drug concentration is based on total drug concentration; therefore, if the free fraction is high because of lower albumin levels, the measured concentration of the drug will underestimate the amount of active drug at the target organ. This is important in assessing blood levels of highly protein-bound drugs such as digoxin, warfarin, theophylline, and phenytoin, which have narrow therapeutic indices.

The rate of drug metabolism by the liver is determined by hepatic function and blood flow. Hepatic mass and functioning hepatocytes decrease with age, and hepatic blood flow is reduced by 0.3% to 1.5% per year after age 25 (Chutka et al. 1995). This results in a substantial reduction in "first-pass" metabolism of a drug in the liver, so more of the active drug remains available. Phase I hepatic metabolism is performed by the microsomal oxidase cytochrome P450 (CYP) system. Initially, these oxidative conversions may produce pharmacologically active metabolites, and subsequent oxidations produce progressively more water-soluble compound that can be excreted by the kidneys and gut. Some of the cytochrome enzymes are affected by aging, most notably CYP 1A2 and CYP 3A4 (Jacobson et al. 2002). The latter is one of the most abundant of the CYP enzymes and is important in the metabolism of a wide variety of drugs (e.g., retroviral agents, antibiotics, antifungals, quinidine, calcium channel blockers, statin drugs, various serotonin reuptake inhibitors, and several antipsychotics, including haloperidol, quetiapine, clozapine, and ziprasidone). The CYP 1A2 enzymes are involved in the metabolism of clozapine, olanzapine, theophylline, and caffeine, whereas CYP 2D6 is involved in the metabolism of many antipsychotics (e.g., risperidone), antidepressants, mood stabilizers, analgesics, and beta-blockers, and does not seem to be affected by age.

Phase II hepatic metabolism involves the conjugation of drugs or their metabolites with glucuronide sulfate or acetyl moieties to produce polar, pharmacologically inactive, hydrophilic compounds that can be excreted. These processes are typically not affected by normal aging, although they may be slowed by malnutrition and extreme old age.

Clearance depends on the removal of a drug from systemic circulation by the liver and kidney. As noted above, age-associated declines in hepatic function and blood flow affect liver clearance, whereas age-associated reductions in renal blood flow and glomerular filtration rate (GFR) affect kidney clearance. Compared with normal younger persons, renal blood flow and GFR are reduced by about 35% to 40%. Thus, clearance of various drugs such as digoxin, gentamicin, procainamide, gabapentin, and lithium that undergo renal elimination are affected by aging.

Pharmacodynamics, which is end-organ responsiveness to medications, is also affected by aging, although it has been much less studied than pharmacokinetic changes. Some of the pharmacodynamic changes noted with aging include reduced density of muscarinic, opioid, and D_2 dopamine receptors; impaired ability to upregulate and downregulate postsynaptic receptors; reduction in most enzyme activities affecting neurotransmitters; and increased or decreased receptor sensitivity, depending on the type of medication (Jacobson et al. 2002). The clinical conclusion is that older persons are more susceptible to the adverse effects of medications, particularly the psychotropic drugs. Among the principal effects, as described by Zubenko and Sunderland (2000), are

- Peripheral anticholinergic effects such as dry mouth, constipation, blurred vision, and urinary retention in males.
- Central nervous system effects (anticholinergic and antihistaminic) such as confusion, sedation, and memory impairment.
- Motor effects such as tremor, impaired gait, extrapyramidal symptoms, falling, and postural instability.
- Cardiovascular effects such as orthostatic hypotension, cardiac conduction delays, and tachycardia.
- Miscellaneous effects such as gastrointestinal disturbances, headache, agitation, sexual dysfunction, hyponatremia, and impaired insulin response.

Finally, because at least 90% of persons age 65 and over take at least one medication daily, and most take two or more (Chutka et al. 1995), it is important to be aware of drug interactions. Potential interactions may be due to effects of one drug on the metabolism of the other so that blood levels of one or both drugs may be raised or lowered, with competition for protein-binding sites thus producing a transient increase in the free concentrations of one or both drugs; or concomitant administration of two drugs with similar side-effect profiles, exacerbating the level of adverse effects. Several key points emerge with respect to the use of medications in older schizophrenic persons, particularly the coadministration of antipsychotic agents and other medications:

- Determine if there are any hepatic, renal, neurological, nutritional, or other medical disorders that are likely to enhance medication side effects.
- Determine if any newly prescribed drug is an inhibitor or inducer of CYP enzymes that are involved with the clearance of the patient's antipsychotic medication.
- Review the side-effect profile of any new medication to be sure that it does not add to the side effects of the patient's antipsychotic medication. For example, the anticholinergic effects of tolterodine (Detrol) may enhance the anticholinergic effects of olanzapine or clozapine.
- It is important to perform baseline and periodic monitoring of electrocardiogram, white cell count, serum sodium, fasting glucose, weight, and vital signs, including blood pressure sitting and standing, due to the propensity of various antipsychotic agents to affect cardiac conduction, induce leukopenia, create insulin resistance and glucose intolerance, cause hyponatremia, and produce orthostatic hypotension. Other drugs that can affect these indices should be used cautiously and may require even more frequent monitoring.

- Monitoring of medication blood levels must take into account low levels of albumin or competition between highly bound drugs. In these instances, the total concentration of the drug (which is the result reported by the laboratory) may decline, although the free drug concentration has not changed. This could result in unnecessary increases in medication dosages or the occurrence of toxicity at seemingly therapeutic doses of the medication.

Health Care Issues

Findings from the PORT study, in which one-sixth of the patients were age 55 and over, indicate that, with the exception of diabetes and hypertension, more than 30% of the schizophrenic patients who reported current physical problems were not receiving treatment for them (Dixon et al. 1999). A variety of patient, physician, and systemic factors have been identified as potential impediments to health care for schizophrenic persons in general. For example, patients may lack insight into a physical condition, have impaired ability to communicate with a physician, or have emotional/behavioral problems that could interfere with the evaluation. Also, physicians may be more apt to conduct inadequate physical examinations, take a poor history, fail to repeat labs or tests as needed, misinterpret physical symptoms as manifestations of psychosis, or passively accept consultative recommendations (Felker et al. 1996). Systemic factors may also affect health care, especially among older schizophrenic persons. Many older persons with schizophrenia receive Medicaid, either alone or with Medicare. However, Medicaid reimbursement, eligibility requirements, and coverage vary widely across the nation, and Medicaid generally lacks the flexibility in choice of provider that may be available with Medicare. Medicaid patients are often relegated to public-sector health programs that are overcrowded and not well equipped to deal with older persons with psychiatric problems. On the other hand, for persons who receive only Medicare, there is virtually no coverage for psychiatric day programs, prescription medications, home attendants, case management, home visits, transportation, and other essential outpatient services. Moreover, outpatient psychiatric treatment requires a 50% copayment. Thus, Medicare copayments for psychiatry continue to be 2.5 times those of other medical specialties, and reimbursable services are heavily weighted toward inpatient care. Of note, outlays for treatment of psychiatric disorders account for 2.5% of Medicare spending, of which over half are to persons under age 65 (Gottlieb 1996).

Despite the dire concerns about inadequate health care for schizophrenic persons, data from the previously cited study of older schizophrenic persons in New York City suggest that the situation may not be so bleak for the geriatric population. Ninety three percent of the sample of 117 outpatients had seen a physician other than a psychiatrist in the past year, and nearly three-quarters had seen their doctor in the past month (C.I. Cohen, unpublished data). The number of visits to nonpsychiatric health providers was actually somewhat greater than for the community comparison group. In addition, one-third of the sample had seen a dentist in the past year, and among women, 28% and 44% reported that in the past year they had received a pap smear and breast examination, respectively. Moreover, the percentages of persons reporting receiving medication for heart disorders, hypertension, or diabetes were 77%, 81%, and 85%, respectively. A combination of factors played a role in patients' seeking out and complying with medical treatment, including the availability of health insurance (Medicare and Medicaid in most instances), easier access to public transportation and ambulette services, wider availability of home attendant services to assist patients and to accompany them to medical visits, and participation in programs that encouraged physical assessments. As noted previously, differences in the availability of services vary from state to state, and New York has a more generous program than most states.

With the expansion of managed care programs for Medicaid and Medicare recipients, a critical issue will be whether schizophrenic persons would be better off in so-called carved-in or carved-out programs (Cohen et al. 2000). The former provide mental health coverage as part of an overall package. The potential advantage is better integration of medical and psychiatric care, and older schizophrenic persons would have greater access to preventive as well as ongoing medical care. The disadvantage is that such programs may underfund psychiatric treatment and attempt to exclude those persons with more severe and persistent mental disorders. The carved-out programs allow for separate coverage for physical health and psychiatric care. The advantage is that such programs, if adequately funded, may allow for more appropriate services for older chronically ill psychiatric patients. The disadvantage is that there is no integration of health and psychiatric services.

At the practical level, the psychiatric clinician may have to employ a variety of strategies to enhance medical care of older schizophrenic persons. First, they should try to ensure that all persons eligible for Medicaid apply for it because it can fill many of the gaps in services not provided by Medicare, such as prescription medication, home care services, day treatment, and psychosocial rehabilitation. In many instances, persons may be eligible for "buy-ins" for Medicaid based on their monthly medical expenditures. Second, clinicians should work with patients to obtain free medications through patient assistance programs offered by most pharmaceutical companies or by enrolling in state-operated prescription programs for seniors (e.g., the Elderly Pharmaceutical Insurance Coverage [EPIC] program in New York). Many of these programs allow eligible persons to have annual incomes of $20,000 to $30,000, and unlike Medicaid, they do not count personal assets. In many communities, public and voluntary health facilities offer care with sliding scales that may include prescription medications, and the VA program is an excellent, low-cost option for eligible veterans.

For older patients who are resistant to seeking formal medical care, there are a number of potential strategies. First, it may be possible to arrange for the services of a primary care doctor, physician's assistant, nurse practitioner, or phlebotomist at a mental health facility, particularly if the patients can be consolidated into a specific time block. Some health services can be conducted at home through mobile health units, local medical laboratories, and the visiting nurse services; the latter can assist with physical therapy in the home, medication monitoring, and home health aides for physical health problems of limited duration. In general, these home health services are covered by Medicare. Finally, psychiatrists may need to serve temporarily as primary care doctors for their older patients until suitable ongoing health care services can be arranged. The extent to which a psychiatrist should serve as a primary care physician remains controversial. Many geropsychiatrists as a matter of practice routinely conduct periodic physical assessments of their patients, and it is not difficult to oversee the management of uncomplicated common medical problems such as hypertension, gastritis, osteoarthritis, or NIDDM.

Issues of Competency

Finally, capacity and competency can be thorny problems in the case of older schizophrenic persons. It should be recalled that *capacity* refers to the opinion of a clinical evaluator concerning a person's functional ability to make independent, authentic decisions about his or her life, whereas *competency* refers to the judgment of the court about such abilities (Grossberg and Zimny 1996). When the person is competent, he or she may create a legal document ("power of attorney") in which someone is designated to act on his or her behalf if the person is not competent to do so. Alternatively, the older person may sign a "health care proxy," which designates someone to act on his or her behalf regarding medical matters and end-of-life decisions. If prior arrangements have not been made, surrogate management arrangements can be established through the use of a representative payee, guardian, or conservator.

Issues of competency are more problematic in older schizophrenic individuals because the demarcation of incapacity becomes murkier. In younger schizophrenic persons, incapacity is typically due to psychotic processes, although substance abuse can confound the etiology of the disturbance. In older schizophrenic persons, in addition to the effects of psychoses, the effects of neuropsychological deficits and medical disorders must be carefully considered. Whereas as many as three-fourths of schizophrenic people evidence some neuropsychological deficits within the first few years of their illness, roughly one-fifth of persons have a very poor long-term outcome with respect to psychopathology and cognition (Davis 2002). In their seventh and eighth decades of life, such persons reach levels of cognitive deficits comparable with persons with moderate to severe Alzheimer's disease, although no Alzheimer's disease neuropathology is present (Davis 2002). In a larger group of schizophrenic persons, as part of the normal aging process there is a modest decline in cognitive functioning (Cohen and Talavera 2000). Because many of these persons also had some mild cognitive deficits at the onset of their illness, this decline in cognitive functioning with age places many older schizophrenic persons at a level comparable with mild to moderate dementia. Moreover, in both groups of schizophrenic persons, undiagnosed or poorly treated medical conditions, increased sensitivity to psychotropics and other medications, adverse drug interactions, small-vessel disease in the brain, sensory impairments, or lack of environmental stimulation and isolation can worsen cognitive status. Thus, older schizophrenic persons often show considerable improvement in their psychopathology, especially positive symptoms, but they remain functionally impaired because of cognitive deficits. Moreover, unlike Alzheimer's disease, in which cognitive decline is more apparent and is appreciable over a few years, cognitive decline in schizophrenia is insidious, and the clinician may not be aware that the patient's cognitive functioning has become grossly abnormal.

Thus, apart from their risk of developing a primary dementia such as Alzheimer's disease or vascular dementia (which is no higher than the risk of their age peers), older schizophrenic persons may develop diminished capacity due to the following: psychoses, cognitive decline, medical or environmental factors. Although any of these factors alone may not reach levels sufficient to affect competency, the potential for several factors to occur in concert may result in more pronounced deficits. This means that the practicing clinician should regularly monitor the cognitive status of the older schizophrenic person (e.g., periodic Mini-Mental State exams); carefully review laboratory results, especially those that may be more likely to affect cognition (e.g., B_{12}, folate, thyroid indices, sodium, glucose, blood levels of lithium and other mood stabilizers); and be vigilant for any drug interactions that might affect cognition. Because they are at increased risk for diminished capacity, middle-aged and elderly schizophrenic patients who are currently competent should be encouraged to complete a health care proxy or to establish a power of attorney.

Conclusion

Schizophrenic persons in general are thought to have worse physical health than their age peers; however, a small body of data suggests that older schizophrenic persons in treatment programs do not have more physical problems than their age peers, although the severity of their medical conditions may be slightly worse. While studies of the general schizophrenic population indicate high rates of undertreatment of medical disorders, data from a study specifically looking at older schizophrenic outpatients found a high proportion were receiving treatment, and greater than 9 in 10 had seen a nonpsychiatric physician in the past year. However, older schizophrenic persons perceive their health as worse than that of their age peers, and this seems to be related to their higher rates of depression and impaired adaptive functioning. Treatment rates in older schizophrenic persons may be higher than in younger schizophrenics because of better insurance (i.e., availability of Medicare as well as Medicaid), as well as treatment programs that encourage regular examinations for older patients. Nevertheless, psychiatrists may need to develop alternative approaches to ensuring health care for older persons, including use of mobile health teams, home phlebotomy, visiting nurse services, and assumption of a primary care role.

In the treatment of older patients with schizophrenia, clinicians must be cognizant of the pharmacokinetic changes associated with aging, the most important of which involve metabolism and clearance of medications. Pharmacodynamic changes associated with aging also result in heightened sensitivity to the potential side effects of medications. Moreover, older persons consume multiple medications, and they are thus more likely to experience adverse effects of drug interactions and are more vulnerable to side effects when they do occur.

Although positive symptoms tend to decline with age, many older schizophrenic persons have appreciable levels of cognitive impairment. Such impairments can be exacerbated by medical illness, side effects of medications, cerebral microvascular disease, environmental understimulation, and psychoses. These cognitive deficits can create thorny problems regarding competency, and clinicians are advised to encourage currently competent middle-aged and elderly schizophrenic patients who are at risk for future cognitive impairment to complete a health care proxy or establish a power of attorney. Because the number of older schizophrenic persons is expected to double over the next 30 years, the paucity of literature available on their health needs and treatment underscores the critical need for longitudinal investigations involving large samples of aging schizophrenic persons that reflects their diverse cultural and economic backgrounds.

References

Allebeck P: Schizophrenia: a life-shortening disease. Schizophr Bull 15: 81–89, 1989

Alstrom CH: Mortality in mental hospitals with special regard to tuberculosis. Acta Psychiatrica et Neurologie suppl no 24, 1942

Baldwin JA: Schizophrenia and physical disease. Psychol Med 9:611–618, 1979

Brown S, Inskip H, Barraclough B: Causes of the excess mortality of schizophrenia. Br J Psychiatry 177: 212–217, 2000

Chutka DS, Evans JM, Fleming KC, et al: Drug prescribing for elderly patients. Mayo Clin Proc 70:685–693, 1995

Cohen CI, Talavera N: Functional impairment in older schizophrenic persons. Am J Geriatr Psychiatry 8:237–244, 2000

Cohen CI, Cohen GD, Blank K, et al: Schizophrenia and older adults. Am J Geriatr Psychiatry 8:19–28, 2000

Davis KL: New insights from early Alzheimer's disease and late-stage schizophrenia. Paper presented at the 15th annual meeting of the American Association of Geriatric Psychiatry, Orlando, FL, February 24–27, 2002

de Leon J, Verghese C, Tracy JI, et al: Polydipsia and water intoxication in psychiatric patients: a review of the epidemiological literature. Biol Psychiatry 35: 408–419, 1994

Dixon L, Postrado L, Delahanty J, et al: The association of medical comorbidity in schizophrenia with poor physical and mental health. J Nerv Ment Dis 187:496–502, 1999

Dixon L, Weiden P, Delahanty J, et al: Prevalence and correlates of diabetes in national schizophrenia samples. Schizophr Bull 26:903–912, 2000

Dynes JB: Cause of death in schizophrenia. Behav Neuropsychiatry 1:12–14, 1969

Eaton WW, Hayward C, Ram R: Schizophrenia and rheumatoid arthritis: a review. Schizophr Res 6:181–192, 1992

Ehrentheil OF: Common disorders rarely found in psychotic patients. Archives of Neurology and Psychiatry 77:178–186, 1957

Ettigi P, Lal S, Friesen HG: Prolactin, phenothiazines, admissions to mental hospitals, and carcinoma of the breast. Lancet 2:266–267, 1973

Felker B, Yazel JJ, Short D: Mortality and medical comorbidity among psychiatric patients: a review. Psychiatr Serv 47:1356–1363, 1996

Fox BH, Howell MA: Cancer risk among psychiatric patients: a hypothesis. Int J Epidemiol 3:207–208, 1974

Goode DJ, Corbett WT, Shey HM, et al: Breast cancer in hospitalized psychiatric patients. Am J Psychiatry 138:804–806, 1981

Gottlieb GL: Financial issues, in Comprehensive Review of Geriatric Psychiatry II, 2nd Edition. Edited by Sadavoy J, Lazarus LW, Jarvik LF, et al. Washington, DC, American Psychiatric Press, 1996, pp 1065–1085

Grossberg GT, Zimny GH: Medical-legal issues, in Comprehensive Review of Geriatric Psychiatry II, 2nd Edition. Edited by Sadavoy J, Lazarus LW, Jarvik LF, et al. Washington, DC, American Psychiatric Press, 1996, pp 1037–1049

Hussar AE: Leading causes of death in institutionalized chronic schizophrenic patients: a study of 1,275 autopsy protocols. J Nerv Ment Dis 142:45–57, 1966

Jacobson SA, Pies RW, Greenblatt DJ: Handbook of Geriatric Psychiatry. Washington, DC, American Psychiatric Publishing, 2002

Jeste DV, Gladsjo JA, Lindamer LA, et al: Medical comorbidity in schizophrenia. Schizophr Bull 22:413–430, 1996

Jos CJ, Evenson RC, Mallya AR: Self-induced water intoxication: a comparison of 34 cases with matched controls. J Clin Psychiatry 47:368–370, 1986

Kovar MG: Health assessment, in The Encyclopedia of Aging, 3rd Edition. Edited by Maddox GL. New York, Springer, 2001, pp 461–464

Krach P: Functional status of older persons with schizophrenia. J Gerontol Nurs 8:21–27, 1993

Lacro JP, Jeste DV: Physical comorbidity and polypharmacy in older psychiatric patients. Biol Psychiatry 36:146–152, 1994

Lipper S, Werman DS: Schizophrenia and intercurrent physical illness: a critical review of the literature. Compr Psychiatry 18:11–22, 1977

Malzberg B: Mortality from cancer among patients with mental disease in the New York Civil State hospitals. Psychiatr Q Suppl 24:73–79, 1950

Marsh CM: Psychiatric presentations of medical illness. J Geriatr Psychiatry 20:181–204, 1997

Mors O, Mortensen PB, Ewald H: A population-based register study of the association between schizophrenia and rheumatoid arthritis. Schizophr Res 40:67–74, 1999

Mortensen PB: Environmental factors modifying cancer risk in schizophrenia. Paper presented at the World Psychiatric Association Symposium, Copenhagen, August 1986

Mortensen PB: The incidence of cancer in schizophrenic patients. J Epidemiol Community Health 43:43–47, 1989

Mortensen PB: Neuroleptic medication and reduced risk of prostate cancer in schizophrenic patients. Acta Psychiatr Scand 85:390–393, 1992

Mortensen PB, Juel K: Mortality and causes of death in schizophrenic patients in Denmark. Acta Psychiatr Scand 81:372–377, 1990

Mortensen PB, Juel K: Mortality and causes of death in first admitted schizophrenic patients. Br J Psychiatry 163:183–189, 1993

Mukherjee S: High prevalence of type II diabetes in schizophrenic patients (abstract). Schizophr Res 15:195, 1995

Mukherjee S, Decina P, Bocola V, et al: Diabetes mellitus in schizophrenic patients. Compr Psychiatry 37: 68–73, 1996

Nissen HA, Spencer KA: The psychogenic problem (endocrine and metabolic) in chronic arthritis. N Engl J Med 214:576–581, 1936

Odegaard O: Mortality in Norwegian mental hospitals 1926–1941. Acta Genetica 2:141–173, 1951

Rappaport MH, Delrahim KK: An abbreviated review of immune abnormalities in schizophrenia. CNS Spectr 6:392–397, 2001

Sabbath JC, Luce RA: Psychosis and bronchial asthma. Psychiatr Q 26:562–576, 1952

Sajatovic M, Popli A, Semple W: Ten-year use of hospital-based services by geriatric veterans with schizophrenia and bipolar disorder. Psychiatr Serv 47:961–965, 1996

Saku M, Tokudome S, Ikeda M, et al: Mortality in psychiatric patients, with a specific focus on cancer mortality associated with schizophrenia. Int J Epidemiol 24:366–372, 1995

Schoos R, Cohen CI: Medical co-morbidity in older schizophrenic persons, in Schizophrenia Into Later Life. Edited by Cohen CI. Washington, DC, American Psychiatric Publishing, 2003

Sheline YI: High prevalence of physical illness in a geriatric psychiatric inpatient population. Gen Hosp Psychiatry 12:396–400, 1990

Tsuang MT, Perkins K, Simpson JC: Physical diseases in schizophrenia and affective disorder. J Clin Psychiatry 44:42–46, 1983

Verbrugge LM, Lepkowski JM, Konkol LL: Levels of disability among U.S. adults with arthritis. J Gerontol B Psychol Sci Soc Sci 46:S71–S83, 1991

Weiner BP, Marvit RC: Schizophrenia in Hawaii: analysis of cohort mortality risk in a multi-ethnic population. Br J Psychiatry 131:497–503, 1977

Wood JB, Evenson RC, Cho DW, et al: Mortality variations among public mental health patients. Acta Psychiatr Scand 72:218–229, 1985

Zubenko GS, Sunderland T: Geriatric psychopharmacology: why does age matter? Harv Rev Psychiatry 7:311–333, 2000

Chapter 9

Substance Use Disorders in Schizophrenia

Alison Netski, M.D.
Christopher Welsh, M.D.
Jonathan M. Meyer, M.D.

Introduction

The co-occurrence of severe mental illness and substance abuse presents complex issues for mental health practitioners, particularly when treating patients with schizophrenia, in whom there is a higher prevalence of substance use disorders than seen in all other psychiatric diagnostic groups, with the sole exception of antisocial personality disorder. Approximately 50% of individuals with schizophrenia will develop substance use disorders at some point during their lives, and about one-half of this group will exhibit current substance abuse or dependence (Cuffel et al. 1994). The abuse of drugs and alcohol by persons with severe mental illness has a wide range of adverse effects on the course of mental illness and psychosocial functioning, including compliance, prognosis, and rates of acute service utilization. This chapter provides a brief overview of the scope of the problem, with a detailed focus on the demographics of substance use, the adverse consequences of the major drugs of abuse in patients with schizophrenia, and the clinical approach to dually diagnosed patients.

Demographics of Substance Use in Patients With Schizophrenia

The proportion of schizophrenia patients suffering from a comorbid drug or alcohol use disorder varies tremendously in published studies, from as low as 10% to as high as 70% (Mueser et al. 1990). The observed range is partially due to variability in the diagnostic criteria employed for schizophrenia, sample demographic characteristics (e.g., male vs. female, urban vs. rural), the types of patient populations studied (e.g., inpatient vs. outpatient), and different criteria for defining drug and alcohol disorders (e.g., DSM-III-R diagnosis, positive urine toxicology screens, rating scales) (Mueser et al. 1990). Although structured clinical interviews have been found to produce the most reliable diagnoses, these are time consuming and expensive due to the need for trained personnel, and therefore are not often used in clinical studies (Mueser et al. 1995). Surveys conducted exclusively in inpatient settings tend to produce higher rates of substance use disorders, in part because persons with dual disorders (i.e., substance use and another major Axis I disorder) are more likely to enter into treatment because exacerbation of either problem may become a focus of clinical attention (Mueser et al. 1995).

The Epidemiologic Catchment Area (ECA) study revealed that 47% of all individuals in the United States with a lifetime diagnosis of schizophrenia or schizophreniform disorder met criteria for some form of substance abuse or dependence (33.7% for alcohol disorder and 27.5% for another drug abuse disorder) (Regier et al. 1990). This figure is comparable with the range of 40%–60% lifetime prevalence gleaned from an analysis of 47 published studies of schizophrenia patients with sample sizes of at least 30 in which the criteria for abuse or dependence were clearly delineated (Cantor-Graae et al. 2001). The authors of this review also found that studies in which more than one method of diagnosis was employed (e.g., chart review plus interview) yielded higher prevalence rates compared with studies that relied on a single method. Regardless of method, in community samples of patients with schizophrenia that are not composed solely of inpatient groups, a figure of approximately 50% lifetime prevalence is found repeatedly. This finding is replicated even from sources outside the United States, such as the recent study combining both structured interview and chart review of 87 patients with schizophrenia in Malmo, Sweden, which noted a lifetime prevalence of any substance use disorder of 48.3% (47.1% for alcohol alone or in combination with other drugs, 26.4% for alcohol only) (Cantor-Graae et al. 2001).

In addition to the lifetime prevalence data, the ECA study found that the odds of having a substance abuse diagnosis were 4.6 times greater for persons with schizophrenia compared with the rest of the population, with the odds of alcohol disorders more than 3 times greater and those of other drug disorders 6 times greater (Regier et al. 1990). Among all substances, nicotine is clearly the most frequently abused agent, with prevalence estimates ranging from 70% to 90%, over 3 times greater than the general population estimate of approximately 25% (Davidson et al. 2001). (See more extensive discussion in Chapter 5, "Nicotine and Tobacco Use in Schizophrenia.") Excluding nicotine use, the ECA study results are consistent with other prevalence studies of schizophrenia demonstrating that alcohol tends to be the most frequently abused agent (20%–60%), followed by cannabis (12%–42%) and cocaine (15%–50%) (Chambers et al. 2001). Use of amphetamines (2%–25%), hallucinogens, opiates, and sedative/hypnotics is less common.

The most consistent findings with regard to demographic characteristics are that those who are younger, were younger at age of schizophrenia onset, or are male are more likely than those who are older and female to abuse drugs or alcohol (Hambrecht and Hafner 2000). It is important to note, however, that evidence is accumulating to document that substance use difficulties among women are not sufficiently recognized, and that women with schizophrenia and comorbid substance disorders are less likely to receive substance abuse treatment (Alexander 1996; Comtois and Ries 1995). The undertreatment of women may lead to unrealistically low prevalence estimates in retrospective chart review studies, yet even in interview studies male gender appears as an independent risk factor after the disparities in gender frequency are controlled for among study participants (Cantor-Graae et al. 2001). There is also evidence from the Malmo, Sweden, cohort and other studies indicating that the onset of substance use in schizophrenia occurs at a younger age in males than in females (Salyers and Mueser 2001).

There are conflicting data regarding the functional capabilities of substance-using patients with schizophrenia compared with non–substance users with severe mental illness. In one of the first studies to examine this issue, Mueser et al. (1990) reported findings on 149 recently hospitalized patients who met DSM-III-R criteria for schizophrenia, schizoaffective disorder, or schizophreniform disorder, and found lower educational levels among the substance-abusing severely mentally ill compared with severely mentally ill patients without substance use disorders. Yet later studies have indicated that substance-using patients with schizophrenia might be more functional than non–substance users. Arndt and colleagues' study of 131 schizophrenia patients with and without comorbid substance use ($n=64$ and 67, respectively) matched for symptomatology and clinical history noted better premorbid adjustment among the so-called pathological substance users (Arndt et al. 1992). In another study, comparing 34 patients with schizophrenia who had histories of substance abuse with 17 patients with schizophrenia who were abstinent (Zisook et al. 1992), the substance abusers were more likely to have been married or gainfully employed.

The most comprehensive attempt to correlate symptomatology and social function with substance use among patients with schizophrenia was performed by Salyers and Mueser (2001), employing 404 patients with a history of recent hospitalization (i.e., prior 3 months) recruited from within a large multicenter psychosocial treatment strategies study. Individuals were ages 18–55, agreed to receive fluphenazine decanoate but not other major psychotropic agents, and received at least three of the monthly assessments of psychiatric symptoms, social functioning, side effects, and substance use over the 3- to 6-month follow-up period. It should be noted that those who were homeless or transient and patients with active ongoing physical dependence (or with suspected drug-induced psychosis but not schizophrenia) were excluded.

In this study, those who consistently reported low or no use of substances scored significantly higher than regular drug or alcohol users on assessments of negative symptoms, particularly the social amotivation and diminished expression scores, although the groups were comparable on ratings of psychotic symptoms (Brief Psychiatric Rating Scale [BPRS]) and distress (Symptom Checklist-90). There were also no significant differences in ratings of tardive dyskinesia, parkinsonism, or akathisia between users and nonusers, although those who reported the greatest frequency of social problems had higher akathisia ratings irrespective of degree of substance use. As one might expect from those who manifest greater negative symptomatology, the low- or no-use group also demonstrated more severe impairment in leisure activities and less frequent social contacts. Although the substance users enjoyed a higher level of social functioning, the drug users in particular reported significantly greater interpersonal problems compared with the low-/no-use group. Interestingly, despite the greater social functional status of substance users, this group had an earlier age of onset for their mental illness and more hospitalizations than the low-/no-use group.

The biological correlate of higher functional status can be seen in work by Scheller-Gilkey and colleagues, who examined differences in magnetic resonance imaging scans for a large sample ($n=176$) of schizophrenia patients. The investigators noted the rate of gross brain abnormalities among both alcohol and drug abusers to be less than half the rate found among patients with no history of alcohol or substance abuse, although this finding did not reach the 0.05 level of statistical significance (Scheller-Gilkey et al. 1999).

Demographic differences exist between urban and rural groups with schizophrenia, especially with regard to housing, and there are also data to suggest that patterns of substance use differ between the two settings. Alcohol use alone or in combination with cannabis is likely to be present in schizophrenia patients living in a rural setting, whereas the use of multiple substances, particularly cocaine, is common in urban settings (Mueser et al. 2001).

Perhaps one of the most important demographic trends recently recognized among the severely mentally ill is the high prevalence of human immunodeficiency virus [HIV], hepatitis B, and hepatitis C (Meyer in press). Whereas the former may be transmitted sexually, hepatitis C in the United States is transmitted primarily by use of shared needles among intravenous drug users. (This topic is covered in detail in Chapter 7, "HIV and Hepatitis C in Patients With Schizophrenia.") Patients with schizophrenia are more likely to engage in high-risk behavior resulting in HIV or hepatitis C infection, yet there is remarkably little in the way of data about the extent of intravenous drug abuse in this disorder. In one large study of mentally ill persons (65% of whom had schizophrenia or schizoaffective disorder), 62.1% of those infected with hepatitis C ($n=145$) reported a lifetime history of intravenous drug abuse (IVDA), whereas only 5.1% of the hepatitis C–negative group ($n=604$) reported a history of IVDA (Rosenberg et al. 2001). Among the HIV-positive persons with severe mental illness, the lifetime prevalence of IVDA was 8.6% compared with 1.4% for the HIV-negative group (Rosenberg et al. 2001). Another, smaller study of 91 schizophrenic patients employing two self-reporting measures found a 22.4% lifetime prevalence of injected drug use; moreover, despite IVDA and high-risk sexual behaviors, 65% reported no concern with HIV infection, and AIDS knowledge was significantly lower among the schizophrenic patients than the control group, particularly among those with long-standing illness and multiple psychiatric admissions (Grassi et al. 1999).

Patterns of Substance Abuse Among Persons With Schizophrenia

Overall, it is clear that substance use disorders in persons diagnosed with schizophrenia occur more frequently than in the general population; however, there is little evidence to suggest that persons with schizophrenia abuse substances for different reasons than the general population. Specifically, the literature demonstrates that patients with schizophrenia do not differentially choose to abuse *specific* drugs to ameliorate *specific* psychic states (e.g., anhedonia). Multiple studies also indicate that patients with schizophrenia do not preferentially abuse certain agents, nor does choice of agent correlate with extent of psychopathology; rather, these individuals use those substances most available and affordable (Cantor-Graae et al. 2001; Chambers et al. 2001; Lambert et al. 1997; Mueser et al. 1992). For the most part, research has also failed to find patterns of drug choice in persons with schizophrenia that differ from groups of patients with other major mental disorders. Thus, although the causes of dysphoria in schizophrenia may be linked to the illness (e.g., neuroleptic side effects, negative symptoms, demoralization), data simply do not support the notion that schizophrenic patients uniquely prefer certain drugs.

Evidence for the hypothesis that patients with schizophrenia do not abuse substances to alleviate certain mental states or medication side effects comes from research focusing on patients' reported reasons for substance use, which suggests that persons with schizophrenia abuse drugs for reasons that are similar to those for persons without schizophrenia (i.e., to get high, to feel better, to escape, and to be less depressed) (Dixon et al. 1991). The research on side effects and substance has generally produced mixed results when investigators examined tardive dyskinesia or other measures of extrapyramidal side effects; however, although Salyers and Mueser (2001) found no correlation between akathisia and extent of substance use, both akathisia and related dysphoria have been found in some studies to be associated with current alcohol use and increased risk of future alcohol use (Duke et al. 1994; Voruganti et al. 1997).

One of the better examples of research into reasons for substance use in schizophrenia is the study by Dervaux and colleagues of 100 patients diagnosed with schizophrenia, whose extent of substance use was assessed by diagnostic interview (Dervaux et al. 2001). Other assessment tools in this study included the Positive and Negative Syndrome Scale (PANSS), self-report measures of impulsivity and sensation seeking, and a self-report measure of anhedonia. Forty-one percent of this cohort met lifetime criteria for substance abuse or dependence, but did not differ from the nonabusing patients with schizophrenia on the basis of ratings of anhedonia, or in symptom severity (as rated by PANSS). Interestingly, this study did not find differences between users and nonusers on the basis of age of first psychiatric contact or number of hospitalizations. Nonetheless, the substance abusers rated significantly higher on the measures of impulsivity and sensation seeking in a manner consistent with nonschizophrenic substance users; moreover, these measures were elevated even among the subgroup reporting only past abuse or dependence, leading the authors to suggest that impulsivity and drug-seeking behavior may not be induced by the use of substances, but rather is an inherent aspect of schizophrenia. It should be noted that some studies have found higher reported rates of depression among substance-using schizophrenics (Hambrecht and Hafner 2000), although others have not replicated this finding (Drake et al. 1989; Mueser et al. 1990).

Other observational data lend credence to the hypothesis that addictive behavior occurs independently as an inherent aspect of the neural abnormalities that contribute to schizophrenia, as opposed to being motivated or driven secondarily by symptoms of the disorder or negative psychic states induced by medication. A review of the literature on the biological basis for substance abuse in schizophrenia noted that some individuals do report symptomatic improvement during substance use, yet others note symptom exacerbation but persist in the use of substances (Chambers et al. 2001). Moreover, self-reports of improvement are often at variance with the clinical observation of symptomatic worsening. In addition, substances of abuse have widely divergent effects on neurotransmitters, weakening the assertion that the concurrent use of agents with opposing effects is intended to ameliorate a specific psychic state.

Another observation suggesting that schizophrenia and addictive behavior are independent manifestations of a common underlying dysregulation of neural circuitry is the finding that use of both drugs and alcohol commonly precedes psychosis, and that 77% of first-episode patients are smokers prior to neuroleptic treatment (Chambers et al. 2001). This relationship between substance use and symptom onset is thus an area of intense scrutiny for those who see the predilection toward psychosis and addictive behavior as independent but parallel processes engendered by common neuropsychiatric deficits.

In the literature review cited earlier, Cantor-Graae and colleagues noted two questions involving schizophrenia and substance use that are not clearly answerable with the current body of data. The first is "the extent to which substance use (especially psychoactive substance use) contributes to the development of schizophrenia, whether as an independent risk factor in itself or by precipitating illness onset in vulnerable individuals" (Cantor-Graae et al. 2001, p. 72).

Because substance use, particularly psychotomimetic agents (e.g., hallucinogens) and stimulants, may increase the likelihood of developing psychosis, investigators have examined this issue to determine the course of substance use in relation to onset of psychosis. To assess the temporal sequence of substance abuse and illness onset, Buhler and colleagues performed a structured interview on 232 first-episode patients with schizophrenia, and then prospectively interviewed and followed another sample of 115 first-episode patients representing 86% of consecutive admissions for admissions in the local area (Buhler et al. 2002). The investigators found that 62% of those with drug abuse and 51% with alcohol abuse began their habit before any signs of the illness were manifest, including prodromal nonpsychotic symptoms. Significantly, there was no correlation found between onset of abuse and onset of psychotic symptoms, although it was noted that the onset of abuse and the psychotic disorder occurred in the same month in 18.2% who abused alcohol and 34.6% who used drugs, implying that there may be a subset of schizophrenia patients whose development of psychotic symptoms were speeded or precipitated by substance use, particularly cannabis use. These data from the combined pools of first-episode patients are similar to those reported for the original group of 232 first-episode patients analyzed separately (Hambrecht and Hafner 2000), in which 27.5% had a cannabis use problem more than 1 year (often more than 5 years) before onset of prodromal schizophrenia symptoms, 34.6% had the onset of symptoms and cannabis use in the same month, and in 37.9% symptoms of schizophrenia preceded substance use. As the genetics of the schizophrenia spectrum are elucidated, the role that substances play in the onset of schizophrenia among individuals with varying biological propensities will become clearer.

Impact of Substance Use Disorders on Course of Illness and Outcomes

The second issue discussed by Cantor-Graae and colleagues is "the degree to which history of substance abuse is associated with a more chronic clinical course of schizophrenia" (p. 72). Although research on the impact of drug and alcohol use on course of illness has produced variable results, the overwhelming weight of evidence points toward substance abuse and dependence having adverse short-term and long-term affects. Overall, persons with schizophrenia who abuse drugs and/or alcohol have more psychotic symptoms and psychotic relapses compared with persons with schizophrenia without substance use disorders (Negrete et al. 1986). One of the first short-term prospective studies in recent-onset schizophrenia patients (Linszen et al. 1994) found that significantly more and earlier psychotic relapses occurred in cannabis abusers. This finding was replicated in a long-term follow-up case-control study of 39 cannabis-abusing schizophrenia patients without other major drug use matched for age, gender, and year of admission with 39 non–cannabis-using schizophrenia control subjects (Caspari 1999). After a mean 68.7 ± 28.3 months of follow-up, the cannabis abusers had a significantly greater hospitalization rate, higher BPRS scores, and greater unemployment.

A larger study of relapse rates was performed in Australia using a sample of 99 recently hospitalized patients, ages 18–65, with schizophrenia or related disorders who were followed prospectively for 4 years (Hunt et al. 2002). Of the 99 entered into the study, 66 were still being followed after 4 years. Demographically, the substance users were more likely to be male, to be younger, and to have a forensic history than nonusers, although there were no differences in age of schizophrenia onset or number of prior hospitalizations. The investigators found that medication-compliant patients who used substances had a median time of 10 months until rehospitalization, compared with 37 months for medication-compliant nonusers. Among medication-noncompliant patients, the survival times to rehospitalization were 5 months for substance users and 10 months for nonusers. Although the medication-noncompliant substance users composed 28.3% of the total study sample, they were responsible for 57% of all psychiatric admissions recorded by study participants, with an average of 1.5 per year. Overall, the substance users had an average of 3.6 admissions over the 4 years compared with 1.1 for nonusers ($P<0.05$) and were significantly more likely to be medication noncompliant (users 67% vs. nonusers 34%, $P<0.05$).

Cocaine and stimulant abuse, due to the direct effects on dopamine, have obviously been linked to exacerbation of psychotic symptoms (Dixon et al. 1990), yet increased severity of positive symptoms is seen in users of all substances. As noted previously, Caspari (1999) found higher BPRS ratings in a long-term case-control study of cannabis abusers, some of whom subsequently also abused alcohol but not cocaine or stimulants. Similarly, Buhler et al. (2002) noted a greater extent of positive symptoms during 5 years of follow-up in a group of 29 first-episode schizophrenic users of various substances compared with matched nonusing control subjects. In particular, hallucinations were present for 1.8 months/year for substance users, compared with 0.6 months/year for nonusers ($P<0.05$). There was also a trend toward fewer negative symptoms among users, which reached statistical significance at the 5-year endpoint ($P< 0.03$).

Violence

Substance use disorders in patients with schizophrenia have been associated with violent behavior toward others, suicide (Barry et al. 1996; Dassori et al. 1990; Drake et al. 1989; Fulwiler et al. 1997), and increased risk for contact with the legal system (Hunt et al. 2002). The association of violence with substance use is not unique to schizophrenia or severe mental illness, and has been observed among patients with other mental disorders (Cuffel et al. 1994; Swartz et al. 1998); moreover, this association between substance use and increased risk for violent behavior among persons with severe mental illness has also been described in patient populations outside of the United States. Rasanen et al. (1998) completed a prospective study in Finland on an 11,017-person unselected birth cohort followed to the age of 26 years, which showed that men with schizophrenia who abused alcohol were 25.2 times more likely to commit violent crimes than men without mental illness, whereas nonalcoholic men with mental illness were only 3.6 times more likely to commit violent crimes than males without any psychiatric diagnosis.

Housing Instability and Homelessness

Comorbid substance use disorders in schizophrenia are consistently associated with increased risk for homelessness among persons with schizophrenia (Drake et al. 1991). In Caton and colleagues' (1994) case-control study comparing 100 indigent men with severe mental illness and homelessness with 100 men with schizophrenia who were not homeless, homeless subjects had significantly higher rates of drug abuse. Studies of innovative service models for the homeless mentally ill have found that persons with substance use comorbidity do not benefit as much from these programs as do the non–substance-using severely mental ill individuals, in part due to the fact that substance-using severely mental ill patients lead a more transient lifestyle. In one study of assertive community treatment for the homeless mentally ill, homeless persons with substance use disorders had more moves during the treatment year than other severely mental ill patients (Holohan et al. 1997).

Medical Consequences of the Most Commonly Abused Substances in Schizophrenia

Alcohol

In the general population, alcohol is the most widely used substance of abuse. Sequelae of ethanol use disorders represent the third leading cause of death in the United States, with an estimated 111,000 deaths per year directly attributable to alcohol ingestion. The most common causes of death in alcohol-related disorders are suicide, cancer, heart disease, and hepatic disease (Schuckit 1999).

The acute action of ethanol in the central nervous system (CNS) derives from two main mechanisms: ethanol facilitates the activation of gamma-aminobutyric acid type A (GABAa) receptors, the main inhibitory neurotransmitter system in the CNS, and inhibits the N-methyl-D-aspartate (NMDA) subtype of glutamate receptors, the main excitatory neurotransmitter receptor system in the CNS. The net effects of GABA are thereby potentiated, leading to sedation, and inhibition of NMDA receptors via allosteric modulation appears to be responsible for the intoxicating effects (Schuckit 1999). Sudden cessation of ethanol use in a chronic, heavy drinker often results in an uncomplicated withdrawal syndrome characterized by mild confusion associated with diaphoresis, tremulousness, and increased heart rate, blood pressure, and temperature, all of which can be blocked by administration of GABA-acting drugs such as benzodiazepines. In about 5%–10% of patients with alcohol dependence, this syndrome may progress to delirium tremens (DTs), which is characterized by significant autonomic instability, marked confusion, disorientation, agitation, tremulousness, and hallucinations (auditory, visual, and tactile). The mortality rate for untreated DTs is approximately 5%. Alcohol withdrawal seizures ("rum fits") may also develop independently of DTs, typically within the first 24–48 hours after cessation of alcohol use (Schuckit 1998).

Alcohol consumption plays a role in both acute and chronic medical illness through a variety of mechanisms, some or all of which may be operative in a specific individual (Schuckit 1998). Repeated exposure may lead to alcoholic hepatitis and eventually cirrhosis, with secondary cognitive impairment via hepatic encephalopathy in advanced cirrhosis due to the accumulation of nitrogenous compounds that are inadequately metabolized by the compromised liver. The cirrhotic changes of the liver are also manifested in impaired synthetic function (e.g., decreased production of clotting factors) and reduced metabolism of exogenous toxins such as medications. In the CNS, prolonged alcohol abuse leads to cerebellar degeneration in about 1% of chronic alcoholics, presenting as unsteady gait and mild nystagmus. These symptoms are irreversible and often accompanied by global cognitive decline from direct or indirect effects of chronic alcohol consumption (e.g., head injury, nutritional deficiency, direct neurotoxicity). Finally, peripheral neuropathy is seen in approximately 5%–15% of alcoholics due to nutritional deficiency and direct toxic effects of alcohol on neuronal axons (Schuckit 1998).

Alcohol abuse increases blood pressure and serum triglycerides, and may lead to cardiomyopathy and arrhythmias via toxic effects on cardiac muscle (Schuckit 1998). During the acute intoxication period, tests for blood alcohol level, serum electrolytes glucose, aspartate transaminase (AST), alanine transaminase (ALT), gamma-glutamyltransferase (GGT), hematocrit, and amylase can be useful. For the chronic alcoholic, additional laboratory values that should be monitored include albumin, red blood cell indices, white blood cell count, platelet count, prothrombin time, hepatitis B and C screening, vitamin B_{12}, and folate.

Cocaine and Amphetamines

Cocaine is derived from the coca plant, native to South America, and is typically insufflated nasally ("snorted"), smoked (in the form of "freebase" or "crack"), or injected intravenously. Amphetamines are analogues of naturally occurring ephedrine and have been abused in various forms since their original synthesis in 1887. Currently, d-methamphetamine ("crystal meth," "meth") is the most popular form of amphetamine abused, and in some areas of the country, such as the West Coast, abuse of methamphetamine is more prevalent than cocaine abuse. Cocaine acts as a competitive blocker of dopamine reuptake in the synaptic cleft, which increases the concentration in the cleft, with resultant activation of dopamine type 1 and 2 receptors. In addition, cocaine increases norepinephrine and serotonin neurotransmission via reuptake inhibition, but these monoamines do not play the dominant role in its CNS effects (Jaffe 1999b). By contrast, amphetamine increases the availability of all synaptic monoamines by stimulating the release of catecholamines, particularly dopamine, from the presynaptic terminals. This effect is especially potent for dopaminergic neurons projecting from the ventral tegmental area to the cerebral cortex and limbic areas, known as the "reward pathway."

Patients with schizophrenia who abuse stimulants experience significant increases in the extent of positive symptoms of their psychosis. In comparison to schizophrenia patients, cocaine-abusing patients without underlying psychotic disorders tend to seek treatment more often for depression and anxiety than for psychosis (Serper et al. 1999). Withdrawal following heavy stimulant use may be associated with significant lethargy and depression and an increased risk for suicide (Gawin and Kleber 1986).

Cocaine and amphetamines have similar health effects based on their similar pharmacological activities that result in increased synaptic dopamine and other monoamines. The resultant sympathomimetic and vasoconstrictive properties of these agents are responsible for many of the acute (e.g., myocardial infarction, cardiac arrhythmias, cerebrovascular accidents, seizures) and chronic (e.g., hypertension) effects of ingestion (Jaffe

1999a). The nasal route of administration can lead to general sinus conges-
tion and septal perforation due to chronic ischemia. The intravenous route
of administration not only increases the transmission risk of HIV and hepatitis B and C viruses, but intravenous and subcutaneous ("skin popping")
use may also result in significant cellulitis, bone and joint infections, en-
docarditis, and renal failure (usually as a result of adulterants to the drug).
Smoking cocaine can exacerbate preexisting asthma or chronic obstructive
pulmonary disease, and can produce specific, fibrotic lung changes known
as "crack lung" (Tashkin 2001). Chronic use of stimulants often results in
significant weight loss due to the anorexic effects of these agents.

Cannabis

Cannabis plants and derived products (e.g., hashish) contain many substances that are believed to have psychoactive properties, although the
most important of these is delta-9-tetrahydrocannabinol (THC). The endogenous cannabis receptor is a member of the G protein–linked family
of anandamide receptors, found in the highest concentration in the basal
ganglia, hippocampus, and cerebellum. In animal studies, activation of the
receptor has an effect on monoamine oxidase and GABA (Chaperon and
Thiebot 1999).

The peak intoxication from smoking cannabis occurs after 10–30 minutes. THC and its metabolites accumulate in fat cells and have a half-life
of approximately 50 hours (Franklin and Frances 1999). In intoxication,
behavioral changes include a heightened sensitivity to external stimuli, de-
realization, impaired motor skills, increased reaction time, and euphoria.
Panic attacks can also be seen in inexperienced users. The drug is usually
smoked, but users may ingest orally (e.g., hashish brownies). Psychosis can
also occur during the intoxication period, evidenced by transient paranoid
ideation and, rarely, frank hallucinations. Subjective reported effects of
acute cannabis intoxication in individuals with schizophrenia include a decrease in anxiety and depression and an increase in suspiciousness (Dixon
et al. 1990). In addition, chronic heavy cannabis use can result in an amo-
tivational syndrome that is described as passivity, decreased drive, diminished goal-directed activity, decreased memory, fatigue, problem-solving
deficits, and apathy that can last for weeks following abstinence. This has
been described by various authors in uncontrolled studies, although con-
troversy still exists regarding the exact nature of the syndrome (Franklin
and Frances 1999).

The deleterious health effects of cannabis are related to route of administration and direct effects on body systems. Cannabis cigarettes ("joints"

or "blunts") have more tar and respiratory irritants than tobacco, and are more carcinogenic to laboratory animals. Long-term use has been found to lead to large airway obstruction. There are also direct inhibitory effects on pulmonary antibacterial mechanisms such as destruction of alveolar macrophages, neutrophils, and lymphocytes. In addition, cannabis can cause variations in heart rate and blood pressure. This can lead to an increase in oxygen consumption and increased risk of myocardial infarction in those with coronary artery disease (Woody and MacFadden 1996).

Substance Use Screening and Treatment

Clearly, case finding remains a priority if patients are to be offered any form of treatment aimed at reduction in substance use. Simply put, clinicians must take the initiative to identify patients who have substance use comorbidity. The first step requires screening and assessment. Most patients will not spontaneously assert that they are using substances. Thus, clinicians must actively seek out this information, with best results achieved by using nonjudgmental forms of inquiry such as "How often have you used…?" instead of "Do you use…?" Given the prevalence of substance use, a high index of suspicion is essential. Clinicians should routinely ask all patients about use of alcohol or other drugs and should continue to inquire on a periodic basis, especially with newer patients, who may be reluctant to discuss substance abuse with a new clinician. Because patients sometimes deny drug use when it is present, a multimodal strategy is optimal, including urine toxicology screens, interviews with collateral sources, records from recent hospitalizations, and consultation with other care providers or family if permitted by the patient.

Once a patient acknowledges using substances, a first step in treatment is to conduct a specialized assessment. In addition to the amount and frequency of substance use, it is critical that clinicians get an understanding of each patient's personal economy of substance use. What benefits and costs does he or she perceive to result from using substances? What are the patient's motivations and expectations? A detailed understanding of patients' perspectives on these questions is critical to engaging them in treatment and helping them to negotiate the phases of treatment to recovery.

Treatment for substance use by people with schizophrenia requires an integrated approach, given the extent to which these problems interact and are interconnected (Hellerstein et al. 2001). Although the deleterious effects of comorbid substance use on relapse rates are clear, the literature on interventions offers little guidance due to the paucity of controlled studies. In a recent article Bennett et al. (2001) noted that only seven studies available in the literature through 1998 employed experimental designs, five of which examined "inpatient care or intensive outpatient case management for serious mentally ill clients (primarily for homeless populations), and are not directly applicable to the treatment of the broader population of people with schizophrenia living in the community" (p. 164). In the remaining two controlled studies of outpatient treatment, one found decreased substance abuse and psychiatric severity among patients who began and remained in treatment over several months. The other semicontrolled study, comparing a 12-step program, behavioral skills training, and intensive case management, found that both skills training and case management were more effective than the 12-step program on several outcome measures, but had minimal effects on substance use. "Interestingly, the behavioral treatment was the most effective even though it was not designed specifically to address substance abuse problems and sessions were only held once per week" (p. 164).

More recent controlled studies of integrated dual-diagnosis treatment have demonstrated the efficacy of this approach. McHugo et al. (1999) showed that programs with high fidelity to dual-diagnosis treatment principles produced markedly greater rates of sobriety than other treatment strategies. After 36 months, patients in high-fidelity programs had a 55% rate of stable remission, whereas only about 15% of patients in low-fidelity programs were in stable remission. In Manchester, UK, Barrowclough et al. conducted a controlled 12-month study comparing outcomes in 18 patients with schizophrenia and substance use disorders employing an integrated approach of motivational interviewing, family interventions (including a family support worker), and cognitive behavior therapy, with outcomes from usual care ($n=12$) (Barrowclough et al. 2001). There was high retention in the integrated-care group (94%), with significant improvements compared with usual care on the Global Assessment of Functioning (GAF) scale, PANSS positive symptom scores, and relapse rates. The benefits of a combined, integrated approach, particularly with respect to retention, are also seen in the results of a randomized controlled study by the Combined Psychiatric and Addictive Disorders Program (COPAD) at Beth Israel Medical Center (New York). The components of the COPAD treatment approach include supportive group substance abuse counseling, a multifaceted educational program (mental illness, psychiatric medications, alcohol and drug abuse, HIV), ongoing assessment of substance use via weekly urine toxicology, encouragement to attend self-help groups, monthly psychiatric medication visits, regular communication with other clinicians involved in the patient's care, and as-needed communication with family members (Hellerstein et al. 2001). After 8 months, 11 of 23 in the COPAD cohort remained in treatment, versus only 6 of 24 usual-care patients.

Bennett and colleagues delineated what they perceive as the necessary qualities of a dual-diagnosis program geared toward patients with schizophrenia in their description of the Behavioral Treatment for Substance Abuse in Schizophrenia (BTSAS) model (Bennett et al. 2001). The special requirements of an effective substance abuse treatment program for the schizophrenia population derive from the findings of low motivation for decreasing substance use (41%–60% depending on the substance[s] abused) in schizophrenia patients, and the cognitive deficits and social skills deficits present in schizophrenia. In creating the BTSAS program, the investigators relied on social skills training, "a behavioral approach for rehabilitation of schizophrenia patients that has been successfully employed for the past 25 years... that employs instruction, modeling, role-playing, and social reinforcement" (p. 165).

The components of BTSAS include monthly motivational interviews to discuss treatment goals; urinalysis, with rewards for abstinence; social skills training, which teaches patients how to refuse offers of drugs; education on the effects of drug use in schizophrenia; and problem-solving and relapse prevention training to help patients cope with urges and high-risk situations. Most skills groups meet twice per week, a similar frequency to the group counseling in COPAD. Recognizing the difficulty that schizophrenia patients have in changing behavior, and that many are abusing multiple substances, the program entails no mandated need to be abstinent or committed to total abstinence to participate; any decrement in use is seen "as a positive step that will reduce patients' overall level of harm" (p. 165) and bring the patient closer to their eventual goal.

Finally, in a discussion of implementing dual-diagnosis programs for substance-abusing patients with schizophrenia, Drake et al. (2001) listed several other critical components for integrated programs, including staged interventions for those at different stages of the recovery process, assertive outreach to engage clients (especially the homeless), the need to maintain a long-term perspective on the chronic and relapsing problems of substance use, and cultural sensitivity. They also noted the barriers that exist in implementing such integrated programs, including administrative issues (policy, programmatic barriers), clinician barriers due to lack of dual-diagnosis training, and consumer barriers due to denial or low motivation. Although the preceding models have not focused on intensive case management, the problems with medication noncompliance, housing, and psychosocial issues associated with substance use often warrant a case management approach, especially for those who are frequent utilizers of inpatient services.

As with all schizophrenia patients, antipsychotic medication is a fundamental aspect of treatment. Although medication-compliant substance users do relapse at higher rates than nonusers, the greatest risk for relapse is with medication-noncompliant substance users. In general, there are no absolute contraindications to the prescription of antipsychotics for schizophrenic patients who are currently using substances, apart from those who are medically compromised (e.g., hepatic disease, HIV), in whom dosage adjustment may be necessary. However, one must use reasonable caution in the use of the more sedating agents in patients abusing alcohol or other CNS depressants (e.g., opiates).

That antipsychotic medication will reduce the likelihood of psychotic relapse even in the presence of ongoing substance use is substantiated by data from the Australian 4-year prospective study (Hunt et al. 2002), yet there are recent studies indicating that the use of atypical antipsychotics might be associated with reductions in substance use. The data are most compelling for clozapine. One 3-year prospective study of 151 dual-diagnosis patients found that 79.0% of clozapine patients ($n=36$) achieved full remission from alcohol use for 6 months or longer, compared with 33.7% for clozapine nonrecipients (Drake et al. 2000). Another retrospective study of 45 dual-diagnosis patients prescribed clozapine noted that 85% decreased their substance use during the course of therapy, with the extent of decrease in abuse corresponding to symptomatic improvement (Zimmet et al. 2000). Promising data in prospective open-label trials have also been published related to risperidone (Smelson et al. 2002) and olanzapine (Littrell et al. 2001) therapy. These agents appear to be safe in the substance-abusing schizophrenia population, as is clozapine, which is both sedating and associated with dose-dependent lowering of the seizure threshold. The approval of a long-acting, water-based injectable form of risperidone in many countries (although this form of risperidone has not yet been approved in the United States as of this writing) also means that the therapeutic advantages of an atypical antipsychotic can be provided to patients poorly compliant with oral medication.

Conclusion

Schizophrenia appears to carry with it the propensity for substance abuse, an independent but parallel process that often precedes by many years the onset of psychotic symptoms. The most commonly abused substances in schizophrenia patients are alcohol, cocaine, and cannabis, with the choice of substance based on affordability and availability, and not on inherent aspects of psychopathology. Because the medical sequelae of abuse are numerous, periodic monitoring of urine toxicology and appropriate laboratory values (depending on the substance[s] abused) should be considered as part of the routine care for schizophrenia patients with established or suspected substance use disorders. Given the likelihood that any schizophrenia patient has a past or ongoing substance use problem, a high index of suspicion must be maintained even with patients who deny or minimize the extent of their substance abuse. The greatest chance for optimizing outcomes and reducing the morbidity of substance abuse comes from identification of patients and enrollment into an integrated dual-diagnosis treatment modality designed specifically for substance-abusing or substance-dependent persons with schizophrenia. Routine screening for and increased recognition of substance use disorders in those with schizophrenia must be considered a standard part of psychiatric and medical care for this population.

References

Alexander MJ: Women with co-occurring addictive and mental disorders: an emerging profile of vulnerability. Am J Orthopsychiatry 66:61–70, 1996

Arndt S, Tyrrell G, Flaum M, et al: Comorbidity of substance abuse and schizophrenia: the role of pre-morbid adjustment. Psychol Med 22:379–388, 1992

Barrowclough C, Haddock G, Tarrier N, et al: Randomized controlled trial of motivational interviewing, cognitive behavior therapy, and family intervention for patients with comorbid schizophrenia and substance use disorders. Am J Psychiatry 158:1706–1713, 2001

Barry KL, Fleming MF, Greenley JR, et al: Characteristics of persons with severe mental illness and substance abuse in rural areas. Psychiatr Serv 47:88–90, 1996

Bennett ME, Bellack AS, Gearon JS: Treating substance abuse in schizophrenia: an initial report. J Subst Abuse Treat 20:163–175, 2001

Buhler B, Hambrecht M, Loffler W, et al: Precipitation and determination of the onset and course of schizophrenia by substance abuse: a retrospective and prospective study of 232 population-based first illness episodes. Schizophr Res 54:243–251, 2002

Cantor-Graae E, Nordstrom LG, McNeil TF: Substance abuse in schizophrenia: a review of the literature and a study of correlates in Sweden. Schizophr Res 48:69–82, 2001

Caspari D: Cannabis and schizophrenia: results of a follow-up study. Eur Arch Psychiatry Clin Neurosci 249:45–49, 1999

Caton CL, Shrout PE, Eagle PF, et al: Risk factors for homelessness among schizophrenic men: a case-control study, Am J Public Health 84:265–270, 1994

Chambers RA, Krystal JH, Self DW: A neurobiological basis for substance abuse comorbidity in schizophrenia. Biol Psychiatry 50:71–83, 2001

Chaperon F, Thiebot MH: Behavioral effects of cannabinoid agents in animals. Crit Rev Neurobiol 13:243–281, 1999

Comtois KA, Ries R: Sex differences in dually diagnosed severely mentally ill clients in dual diagnosis outpatient treatment. Am J Addict 4:245–253, 1995

Cuffel BJ, Shumway M, Chouljioa TL, et al: A longitudinal study of substance use and community violence in schizophrenia. J Nerv Ment Dis 182:704–708, 1994

Dassori AM, Mezzich JE, Keshavan M: Suicidal indicators in schizophrenia. Acta Psychiatr Scand 81:409–413, 1990

Davidson S, Judd F, Jolley D, et al: Cardiovascular risk factors for people with mental illness. Aust N Z J Psychiatry 35:196–202, 2001

Dervaux A, Bayle FJ, Laqueille X, et al: Is substance abuse in schizophrenia related to impulsivity, sensation seeking, or anhedonia? Am J Psychiatry 158:492–494, 2001

Dixon L, Haas G, Weiden PJ, et al: Acute effects of drug abuse in schizophrenic patients: clinical observations and patients' self-reports. Schizophr Bull 16:69–79, 1990

Dixon L, Haas G, Weiden PJ, et al: Drug abuse in schizophrenic patients: clinical correlates and reasons for use. Am J Psychiatry 148:224–230, 1991

Drake RE, Osher FC, Wallach MA: Alcohol use and abuse in schizophrenia: a prospective community study. J Nerv Ment Dis 77:408–414, 1989

Drake RE, Osher FC, Wallach MA: Homelessness and dual diagnosis. Am Psychol 46:1149–1158, 1991

Drake RE, Xie H, McHugo GJ, et al: The effects of clozapine on alcohol and drug use disorders among patients with schizophrenia. Schizophr Bull 26:441–449, 2000

Drake RE, Essock SM, Shaner A, et al: Implementing dual diagnosis services for clients with severe mental illness. Psychiatr Serv 52:469–476, 2001

Duke PJ, Pantelis C, Barnes TRE: South Westminster schizophrenia survey: alcohol use and its relationship to symptoms, tardive dyskinesia and illness onset. Br J Psychiatry 164:630–636, 1994

Franklin JE, Frances RF: Alcohol and other psychoactive substance use disorders, in Textbook of Psychiatry, 3rd Edition. Edited by Hales RE, Yudofsky SC, Talbott JA. Washington, DC, American Psychiatric Press, 1999, pp 363–423

Fulwiler C, Grossman H, Forbes C, et al: Early onset substance abuse and community violence by outpatients with chronic mental illness. Psychiatr Serv 48:1181–1185, 1997

Gawin F, Kleber H: Abstinence symptomatology and psychiatric diagnosis in cocaine abusers. Arch Gen Psychiatry 43:107–133, 1986

Grassi L, Pavanati M, Cardelli R, et al: HIV-risk behaviour and knowledge about HIV/AIDS among patients with schizophrenia. Psychol Med 29:171–179, 1999

Hambrecht M, Hafner H: Cannabis, vulnerability, and the onset of schizophrenia: an epidemiological perspective. Aust N Z J Psychiatry 34:468–475, 2000

Hellerstein DJ, Rosenthal RN, Miner CR: Integrating services for schizophrenia and substance abuse. Psychiatr Q 72:291–306, 2001

Holohan N, Dixon L, Drauss N: Outcomes of housing in persons with mental illness and substance use disorders. Poster presented at the 150th annual meeting of the American Psychiatric Association, May 19, 1997, San Diego, CA

Hunt GE, Bergen J, Bashir M: Medication compliance and comorbid substance abuse in schizophrenia: impact on community survival 4 years after a relapse. Schizophr Res 54:253–264, 2002

Jaffe JH: Amphetamine (or amphetamine-like)-related disorders, in Comprehensive Textbook of Psychiatry, 7th Edition. Edited by Sadock BJ, Sadock VA. New York, Lippincott Williams & Wilkins, 1999a, pp 971–981

Jaffe JH: Cocaine-related disorders, in Comprehensive Textbook of Psychiatry, 7th Edition. Edited by Sadock BJ, Sadock VA. New York, Lippincott Williams & Wilkins, 1999b, pp 999–1014

Lambert M, Haasen C, Mass R, et al: [Consumption patterns and motivation for use of addictive drugs in schizophrenic patients] (German). Psychiatr Prax 24:185–189, 1997

Linszen DH, Dingemans PM, Lenior ME: Cannabis abuse and the course of recent-onset schizophrenic disorders. Arch Gen Psychiatry 51:273–279, 1994

Littrell KH, Petty RG, Hilligoss NM, et al: Olanzapine treatment for patients with schizophrenia and substance abuse. J Subst Abuse Treat 21:217–221, 2001

McHugo GJ, Drake RE, Teague GB, et al: Fidelity to assertive community treatment and client outcomes in the New Hampshire Dual Diagnosis study. Psychiatr Serv 50:818–824, 1999

Meyer JM: Prevalence of hepatitis A, hepatitis B and HIV among hepatitis C seropositive state hospital patients: results from Oregon State Hospital. J Clin Psychiatry (in press)

Mueser KT, Yarnold PR, Levinson DF, et al: Prevalence of substance abuse in schizophrenia: demographic and clinical correlates. Schizophr Bull 16:31–56, 1990

Mueser KT, Yarnold PR, Bellack AS: Diagnostic and demographic correlates of substance abuse in schizophrenia and major affective disorder. Acta Psychiatr Scand 85:48–55, 1992

Mueser KT, Bennett M, Kushner MG: Epidemiology of substance use disorders among persons with chronic mental illness, in Double Jeopardy: Chronic Mental Illness and Substance Use Disorders. Edited by Lehman AF, Dixon LB. Chur, Switzerland, Harwood Academic, 1995, pp 9–26

Mueser KT, Essock SM, Drake RE, et al: Rural and urban differences in patients with a dual diagnosis. Schizophr Res 48:93–107, 2001

Negrete JC, Werner PK, Doublas DE, et al: Cannabis affects the severity of schizophrenic symptoms: results of a clinical survey. Psychol Med 16:515–520, 1986

Rasanen P, Tiihonen J, Isohanni M, et al: Schizophrenia, alcohol abuse, and violent behavior: a 26-year follow-up study of an unselected birth cohort. Schizophr Bull 24:437–441, 1998

Regier DA, Farmer ME, Rae DS, et al: Comorbidity of mental disorders with alcohol and other drug abuse: results from the Epidemiologic Catchment Area (ECA) study. JAMA 264:2511–2518, 1990

Rosenberg SD, Goodman LA, Osher FC, et al: Prevalence of HIV, hepatitis B, and hepatitis C in people with severe mental illness. Am J Public Health 91:31–37, 2001

Salyers MP, Mueser KT: Social functioning, psychopathology, and medication side effects in relation to substance use and abuse in schizophrenia. Schizophr Res 48:109–123, 2001

Scheller-Gilkey G, Lewine RR, Caudle J, et al: Schizophrenia, substance use, and brain morphology. Schizophr Res 35:113–120, 1999

Schuckit MA: Alcohol and alcoholism, in Harrison's Principles of Internal Medicine, 14th Edition. Edited by Fauci AS, Braunwald E, Isselbacher KJ, et al. New York, McGraw-Hill, 1998, pp 2503–2508

Schuckit MA: Alcohol-related disorders, in Comprehensive Textbook of Psychiatry, 7th Edition. Edited by Sadock BJ, Sadock VA. New York, Lippincott Williams & Wilkins, 1999, pp 953–970

Serper MR, Chou JCY, Allen MH, et al: Symptomatic overlap of cocaine intoxication and acute schizophrenia at emergency presentation. Schizophr Bull 25:387–394, 1999

Smelson DA, Losonczy MF, Davis CW, et al: Risperidone decreases craving and relapses in individuals with schizophrenia and cocaine dependence. Can J Psychiatry 47:671–675, 2002

Swartz MS, Swanson JW, Hiday VA, et al: Violence and severe mental illness: the effects of substance abuse and nonadherence to medication. Am J Psychiatry 155:226–231, 1998

Tashkin D: Airway effects of marijuana, cocaine, and other inhaled illicit agents. Curr Opin Pulm Med 7:143–161, 2001

Voruganti LNP, Heslegrave RJ, Awad AG: Neuroleptic dysphoria may be the missing link between schizophrenia and substance abuse. J Nerv Ment Dis 185:463–465, 1997

Woody G, MacFadden W: Cannabis-related disorders, in Substance Abuse: A Comprehensive Textbook, 3rd Edition. Edited by Lowinson J, Ruiz P, Millman J, et al. Baltimore, MD, Williams & Wilkins, 1996, pp 810–817

Zimmet SV, Strous RD, Burgess ES, et al: Effects of clozapine on substance use in patients with schizophrenia and schizoaffective disorder: a retrospective survey. J Clin Psychopharmacol 20:94–98, 2000

Zisook S, Heaton R, Moranville J, et al: Past substance abuse and clinical course of schizophrenia. Am J Psychiatry 149:552–553, 1992

Chapter 10

Neurological Comorbidity and Features in Schizophrenia

Theo C. Manschreck, M.D., M.P.H.
Lili C. Kopala, M.D., F.R.C.P.C.
William G. Honer, M.D., F.R.C.P.C.

Introduction

From its earliest descriptions, the group of disorders we designate as schizophrenia has been associated with various neurological manifestations (Nasrallah and Weinberger 1986). In some cases, this has been due to co-occurrence with acquired disorders that have neurological features at rates above those in the general population. Such disorders include alcohol and other substance abuse, head injury, and epilepsy. In other cases the neurological findings have included disturbances of movement, minor physical anomalies, deviations in handedness and lateralization of functions, nonlocalizing neurological signs, eye tracking disturbances, and cognitive deficits. The significance of these findings is not fully understood, but they are considered to be an inherent part of the disorder and occur frequently but not uniquely in schizophrenic patients.

As if the task of understanding neurological aspects of schizophrenia were not already complicated, another issue must be considered. The idiopathic form of this disorder, characterized by the DSM-IV-TR criteria (American Psychiatric Association 2000), is a syndrome. This syndrome, despite its narrow definition, encompasses a remarkable variety of clinical presentations. With the development of modern medicine, various disease entities with clearly identifiable causes or pathologies have been identified that overlap with this syndrome, such as Parkinson's disease, Huntington's disease, Wilson's disease, and temporal lobe epilepsy. These disorders mimic some aspects of schizophrenia, although they are clearly distinguishable from the idiopathic condition.

In short, neurological features may have various forms of association with schizophrenia: they may be an intrinsic part of schizophrenia, they may be a reflection of other (comorbid) diseases that complicate the clinical picture, or they may be characteristics of specific diseases not yet distinguished from schizophrenia.

The purpose of this chapter is to review the comorbid neurological aspects of schizophrenia. From a scientific perspective, the purpose of this chapter is to achieve a better understanding of the nature of comorbid conditions and features as potential clues to pathogenesis and even etiology in schizophrenia. From a clinical perspective, the purpose is to create a better understanding of the complexities of the clinical picture in schizophrenia to inform treatment strategy and planning.

Comorbid Disorders

Having a diagnosis of schizophrenia provides no reduction in risk for the vast majority of medical and psychiatric disorders. One expects, then, to see similar incidence and prevalence rates for these disorders as found in the general population. Strikingly, however, certain neurological conditions occur with greater frequency among patients with schizophrenia than in the general population.

Mental Retardation

Cognitive disturbance is a central feature of schizophrenia, with evidence suggesting that there is a modest reduction in IQ during the early stages of the condition. Overall, there is a higher frequency of schizophrenia among the mentally retarded (MR) and learning disabled, who develop this condition approximately three times more frequently than the general population (Turner 1989). A recent controlled magnetic resonance imaging study (Sanderson et al. 1999) of patients with comorbid schizophrenia and MR, MR alone, or schizophrenia alone compared with normal control subjects found that the scans of those with both disorders were similar to those of the schizophrenia alone group in terms of general structures and the structure of the amygdala-hippocampus. The amygdala-hippocampus was significantly smaller bilaterally than that in control subjects, whereas in MR patients without schizophrenia the amygdala-hippocampal complexes were larger. The authors suggested that the higher frequency of schizophrenia in the MR population is due to the tendency of schizophrenia patients to develop cognitive deficits, and they also proposed that within the MR population there may be individuals whose cognitive deficits result from undiagnosed schizophrenia.

In a subsequent study, Sanderson et al. (2001) found that small amygdala-hippocampal size was associated with a history of central nervous system injury, especially meningitis. These findings provide support for the view that cognitive impairment and comorbid psychosis may result from a common cause, such as meningitis or obstetric complication, possibly interacting with other risk factors, such as family history. O'Dwyer (1997) reported that individuals with intellectual disability who develop schizophrenia have significantly higher rates of maternal pregnancy and birth complications than control subjects.

Patients with comorbid schizophrenia and low IQ may present complex management problems. They require longer hospitalizations than those with schizophrenia alone and are more likely to have a history of epilepsy, negative symptoms, and impairment of episodic memory. Negative symptoms and memory problems are difficult to treat and may contribute to poor adherence to treatment (Doody et al. 1998). At discharge these patients often require a high level of community support due to poorer social support from their families, possibly because of familial learning disability or schizophrenia.

Epilepsy

Patients with epilepsy develop psychosis or schizophrenia at rates exceeding those expected if the two disorders were independent (Mendez et al. 1993; Trimble 1991). Conversely, patients with schizophrenia are more prone to seizures than the general population. The excess in vulnerability may result from the neuropathological changes of schizophrenia itself or the secondary effects of the illness, which include exposure to seizure threshold–lowering medication. One possible common factor is neurodevelopmental abnormalities involving the mesial temporal lobe (Hyde and Weinberger 1997). The chronic interictal psychosis of temporal lobe epilepsy (TLE; i.e., complex partial seizure disorder) at times resembles schizophrenia phenomenologically (Slater et al. 1963). Better preservation of affect, memory impairment, visual hallucinosis, mystical experiences, and mood swings are believed to be more common in TLE with interictal psychosis than in schizophrenia. Also, mean age at onset of TLE is about 30 years (Onuma et al. 1991; Slater et al. 1963). Risk factors include severe and intractable epilepsy, epilepsy of early onset, secondary generalization of seizures, certain anticonvulsant drugs, and temporal lobectomy (Sachdev 1998).

Traumatic Brain Injury

Schizophrenic patients, perhaps because of clumsiness, distractibility, poor coordination, or poor judgment, are subject to various forms of traumatic insult, but there may be other connections. The impact of traumatic brain injury (TBI) on a person's functioning is, of course, related to the extent and type of injury sustained, yet TBI can mimic the features of schizophrenia, making exact diagnosis difficult. Schizophrenia following TBI could be a phenocopy of schizophrenia or the consequence of gene–environment interaction, or the association of a TBI event and schizophrenia could be spurious if those predisposed to schizophrenia have greater trauma for other reasons. Malaspina et al. (2001) investigated the relationship between traumatic brain injury and psychiatric diagnoses in a large group of subjects from families with at least two biologically related first-degree relatives with schizophrenia, schizoaffective disorder, or bipolar disorder. Rates of TBI were significantly higher for those with schizophrenia (19.6% in the schizophrenia pedigree, 4.5% in the bipolar pedigree) than for those with no mental illness. Multivariate analysis of within-pedigree data showed that mental illness was related to traumatic brain injury only in the schizophrenia pedigrees. Members of schizophrenia pedigrees also failed to show the typical greater likelihood of TBI in males compared with females—a gender difference that was present among schizophrenia subjects from the bipolar pedigrees.

Alcohol and Other Substance Abuse Disorders

Substance abuse disorders complicate schizophrenia at rates that exceed those found in the general population. The Epidemiologic Catchment Area study (Regier et al. 1990) found the rate of comorbid substance abuse as 47% in schizophrenia. Alcohol accounted for 34% of this estimated rate, a figure substantially higher than that for the general population (14%). Another recent investigation concluded that individuals with schizophrenia report rates of 16% for lifetime nonalcohol substance abuse (Duke et al. 2001). The most commonly abused substances include marijuana, stimulants, hallucinogens, opiates, and anticholinergics, and abuse was concentrated in males younger than 36 years. The suggested source of this increased vulnerability to addictive behaviors among schizophrenic patients is disturbance in the neural circuitry mediating drug desire and reinforcement. Chambers et al. (2001) argued that abnormalities in the hippocampal formation and frontal cortex (leading to disturbed dopamine and glutamate signaling in the nucleus accumbens) facilitate the positive reinforcing effects of drug reward and reduce inhibitory controls over drug-seeking behavior. See Chapter 9, "Substance Use Disorders in Schizophrenia," for a more complete discussion.

Neurological Features Considered Part of Schizophrenia

Movement Disorders

Pre-antipsychotic Era

Motor abnormalities in severe mental disorders have long been observed and commented on, often with excellent descriptions (Berrios 1993; Bleuler 1911/1950; Kahlbaum 1874/1973; Kraepelin 1919; Manschreck 1986; Rogers 1992). These abnormalities fall into various categories, including posture, gait, and voluntary and involuntary motor movements (Table 10–1).

Kahlbaum (1874/1973), for example, described psychotic patients presenting with catatonia as a distinct syndrome categorized as belonging to a severe, deteriorating type of psychotic illness. The latter was referred to as "dementia praecox," by Kraepelin (1919) and renamed "schizophrenia" by Bleuler (1911/1950).

Not only did early reports identify motor abnormalities in schizophrenia, but case records from the early era have enriched understanding of their relationship to schizophrenia. For example, Kraepelin (1919) described features in dementia praecox indistinguishable from contemporary accounts of tardive dyskinesia (TD; Crow et al. 1982, 1983). Turner (1992) examined casebooks from Ticehurst House Asylum from 1845 to 1890. He counted movement abnormalities (e.g., "ugly grimaces, constant fidgeting, extraordinary attitudes, jerking") when they were clearly re-

Table 10–1.   Abnormalities of spontaneous motor behavior in schizophrenia

Decreased motor activity	Increased motor activity	Postural disturbance
Retardation	Restlessness	Rigidity
Poverty of movement	Excitement	Catalepsy
Stupor	Tremor	Clumsiness
Posturing	Stereotypies/mannerisms	
Motor blocking	Perseverative movements	
Cooperation	Impulsive movements	
Opposition	Mannerisms	
Automatic obedience		
Negativism		
Ambitendency		

corded and unambiguously present. Separately he estimated the probable diagnoses of the cohort using standardized criteria and characterized outcome associated with the presence of motor abnormalities. The findings are instructive. Well before the advent of neuroleptic treatment, abnormal movements were recognized as being associated with mental disorder. These movements were particularly concentrated among patients with diagnoses of schizophrenia and, in striking contrast, largely absent among patients with mood and other brain disorders. Far from being incidental findings, these features were associated with a poorer prognosis and limited social recovery.

Abnormal Voluntary Movements

Although voluntary movement disorders have not been as extensively studied as involuntary movement disorders, data do exist, such as those generated by Manschreck et al. (1982) in their investigation of abnormal voluntary movements in schizophrenic subjects and mood-disordered patient control subjects. The assessment included a 1-hour examination of spontaneous motor activity, examination of simple and complex motor tasks, and evaluation of medication side effects. The findings indicated that 36 of 37 schizophrenic subjects showed disturbed voluntary movements, whereas mood-disordered subjects showed less frequent and less severe disturbances. These were voluntary motor disturbances and not associated with evidence of medication effects. Indeed, antipsychotic medication had a marginally positive impact in reducing the occurrence of such movements, which did not resemble the forms of disturbance characteristic of drug-induced motor effects. These voluntary disturbances fell into three general categories: disruption in the smoothness and coordination of movements, intermittent repetitive movements (e.g., stereotypies), and disturbances in performing sequential actions. These abnormalities were frequent but seldom dramatic in their presentation, and could easily be missed without careful examination. Certain unusual catatonic behaviors, for example, were not observed; on the other hand, stereotyped and manneristic behaviors were common. These results have been replicated (Heinrichs and Buchanan 1988; Manschreck and Ames 1984) and demonstrate the presence of intrinsic voluntary motor abnormality in schizophrenia.

Abnormal Involuntary Movements

In recent years, there have been systematic attempts to characterize abnormal involuntary movements presumed to be intrinsic to schizophrenia. Kraepelin observed that some patients with psychosis had fixed facial expression and slow shuffling movements reminiscent of Parkinson's disease (Crow et al. 1982, 1983) and described features in dementia praecox indistinguishable from contemporary accounts of TD.

Whereas Kahlbaum conceptualized catatonia as a brain disorder, Bleuler believed that all motor symptoms of schizophrenia were in some way related to the psychic factors (Arieti 1972); however, following the epidemic of influenza in the second decade of the twentieth century, which resulted in large numbers of cases of encephalitis lethargica, there was further discourse on the possibility that psychotic symptoms seen in psychiatric disorders and motor dysfunction both arose from abnormal brain function (Dretler 1935; Steck 1926/1927).

When TD was initially described in the 1950s, there was considerable debate about the origins of these movements. For example, some authors suggested that these were stereotypic, whereas others described them as choreiform (Degwitz 1969; Fahn 1983; Klawans 1983). Indeed, there was much discussion about what constituted mannerisms, stereotypies, dyskinetic movements, dystonia, and the parkinsonian symptoms of tremor and rigidity (Rogers 1985). Pertinent to these discussions, Rogers (1985) reported on a population of outpatients who had received a diagnosis of severe psychiatric illness (the majority of them with schizophrenia) and who were initially hospitalized before the introduction of neuroleptic medications (1907–1955). In the process of reviewing their charts, Rogers noted that although these patients were not selected by diagnosis, nearly all met the current criteria for a diagnosis of schizophrenia. In this neuroleptic-naïve population, abnormalities of virtually every aspect of motor function were described (see Table 10–2).

Table 10–2. Comparison of movement disorders among hospitalized schizophrenic patients and those with mental handicaps in the pre-antipsychotic era

Motor disorder	Schizophrenia group (%)				Mental handicap group (n=99) (%)
	Whole group (n=100)	1907–1926 (n=34)	1927–1935 (n=33)	1936–1955 (n=33)	
Speech production	92	94	97	88	85
Activity	84	88	94	70	39
Purposive movement	83	85	79	85	97
Facial movements or postures	77	85	67	79	52
Head, trunk, or limb movements	71	62	76	76	32
Posture	50	50	45	56	62
Eye movements	28	29	24	30	25
Tone	14	21	6	15	54
Gait	10	15	12	3	71
Blinking	5	3	0	12	12

Source. Adapted from Rogers (1985, 1991).

Table 10–3.   Association of current motor disorder with neuroleptic medication status

Motor disorder	Whole group (n=100)	Medication status[a] (%)					
		A (n=43)	B (n=12)	C (n=12)	D (n=12)	E (n=13)	F (n=8)
Purposive movement	97	100	92	92	100	100	88
Speech production	95	98	92	100	83	100	88
Posture	86	88	83	92	67	100	75
Tone	85	93	92	58	75	100	75
Facial movements or postures	74	81	83	58	75	62	63
Head, trunk, or limb movements	67	67	75	83	58	69	38
Activity	64	74	67	67	50	46	50
Stride or associated movements	48	49	42	25	50	62	63
Eye movements	48	50	17	58	42	46	50
Blinking	38	39	67	33	42	23	38

[a]Group A: currently receiving neuroleptic medication
Group B: no medication for 1 month
Group C: no medication for 1 year
Group D: no medication for 5 years
Group E: no medication for 15 years
Group F: never medicated

Source.   Adapted from Rogers (1985).

For these patients, motor dysfunction was as prominent a part of their illness as were their psychotic symptoms and functional disability. Rogers himself conceded that attempting to sort out what was functional and related to psychosis versus what was a neurological manifestation became superfluous if severe psychiatric disorders themselves were viewed as neurological conditions.

The introduction of antipsychotic or neuroleptic medications in the 1950s shifted the focus of attention from the existing motor dysfunction to neuroleptic-induced extrapyramidal signs and symptoms (Manschreck 1986). Chlorpromazine, the first neuroleptic to be widely used, appeared to worsen motor function. In this regard, the term *neuroleptic* actually refers to a substance that produces symptoms resembling those of diseases of the nervous system (Taber's 1981). Specifically, the reference was to Parkinson's disease. Table 10–3 indicates the percentages of patients in the sample Rogers studied who had motor disorders in relation to neuroleptic medications (Rogers 1985). Although those patients who were on active medication had a tendency toward greater prevalence of motor abnormalities, these abnormalities are still seen with high frequency among the never-medicated patients with schizophrenia.

As part of resurgent interest in the evaluation of patients with a first episode of schizophrenia or related psychotic disorder, various aspects of motor dysfunction have been studied prior to any treatment with antipsychotic medication (Browne et al. 2000). In part, this is related to the fact that motor abnormalities clearly predate exposure to neuroleptic medication. Furthermore, it may be possible to correct or ameliorate some aspects of abnormal motor function if patients are treated with one of the newer, second-generation or atypical, antipsychotic medications (Kopala et al. 1998; Whitehorn and Kopala in submission).

Extrapyramidal signs and symptoms are sometimes divided into categories, which include parkinsonism, dystonia, dyskinesia, and akathisia. These signs and the most commonly used clinical and research rating scales are outlined next.

- **Parkinsonism:** Bradykinesia (difficulty initiating movements), rigidity, abnormal gait and posture, tremor, sialorrhea, postural instability, diminished expressive automatic movements, masked facies, low monotonic speech. *Rating scales:* Simpson-Angus Scale (SAS; Simpson and Angus 1970), Extrapyramidal Symptom Rating Scale (ESRS).
- **Dystonia:** Sustained increase in muscle tone resulting in abnormal posture. *Rating scales:* SAS, ESRS.
- **Dyskinesia:** Involuntary movements in any muscle groups. *Rating scales:* Abnormal Involuntary Movement Scale (AIMS), ESRS.

- **Akathisia:** Objective observation of inability to remain still, subjective experience of restlessness and dysphoria. *Rating scale:* Barnes Akathisia Scale (BAS; Barnes 1989).

In reviewing the first-episode data, it becomes clear that a variety of different rating scales have been used to quantify these abnormalities, and that some studies include a heterogeneous sample of young individuals who have been ill for relatively short periods of time and more chronically ill subjects, some of whom were never treated (Fenton 2000). Thus, as can be seen from Table 10–4, there was considerable variability in these studies in the prevalence of parkinsonism, dystonia, and dyskinesia, which may well be related to the heterogeneity and small sample sizes. Nonetheless, it is worth noting that with specific reference to parkinsonian signs, tremor was relatively rare compared with bradykinesia and rigidity.

Newer Findings on Involuntary Movements

As mentioned previously, the historical (and we would argue ongoing) nosological confusion between what is psychiatric versus neurological was evident in many of the studies reviewed (Berrios and Chen 1993; Lund et al. 1991; Rogers 1985). For example, Peralta et al. (2000) attempted to differentiate between the negative symptoms of schizophrenia and parkinsonism. This research group in fact documented a significant correlation between the severity of negative symptoms and the severity of akinetic but not hyperkinetic parkinsonism. An important finding from their study was that 19% of neuroleptic-naïve patients had a parkinsonian syndrome at admission. This number increased to 32% at discharge, after patients were treated with neuroleptic medications, despite the fact that most of the patients (39 of 49) received treatment with so-called new or second-generation antipsychotics, which are believed to produce fewer and less prominent extrapyramidal symptoms compared with typical or first-generation antipsychotics (Leucht et al. 1999). Caligiuri et al. (1993) compared 24 neuroleptic-naïve schizophrenic patients and 24 age- and gender-matched comparison subjects. They found that 29% of the schizophrenic patients had rigidity and 37% had tremor with the use of instrumental measures, in contrast to 4% and none, respectively, of the normal comparison group. The schizophrenic patients also exhibited greater right-side than left-side parkinsonism. Nonetheless, Caligiuri did not find such a relationship between the severity of negative symptoms and the severity of akinetic parkinsonism. Subsequently, our group (Kopala et al. 1998) reported on a sample of neuroleptic-naïve young patients who had extrapyramidal signs and symptoms prior to any treatment. The subgroup with abnormal motor

Table 10–4. Selected studies of extrapyramidal disorder prevalence in never-treated first-episode schizophrenia

	n	Prevalence of parkinsonism (%)							Scale used
		Overall	Rigidity	Bradykinesia	Tremor	Akathisia	Dyskinesia	Dystonia	
Chorfi and Moussaoui (1985) (M=44, F=6)	50						2		AIMS
Caligiuri et al. (1993) (M=20, F=4)	24	21	21	13	0				SAS
Chatterjee et al. (1995) (M=47, F=42)	89	17	7	14	3	6	1		SAS
Fenn et al. (1996) (M=19, F=3)	22	18					14		Hans Rating Scale
Kopala et al. (1998) (M=17, F=5)	32	28	22		3		0	17	ESRS
Gervin et al. (1998) (M=50, F=29)	49						8		AIMS
Puri et al. (1999) (M=18, F=9)	27	4					4		Modified Rogers Scale
Peralta et al. (2000) (M=33, F=14)	49	19							SAS

Note.   AIMS = Abnormal Involuntary Movement Scale; SAS = Simpson-Angus Rating Scale; ESRS = Extrapyramidal Symptom Rating Scale.

Source.   Adapted from Honer et al. (2002).

function had more prominent negative symptoms of psychosis. Chatterjee et al. (1995) reported similar associations between abnormal motor function and negative symptoms. The implication from most of these studies is that abnormalities in brain organization resulted in these two features of the disorder, namely, negativity and akinesis.

To date, studies that attempted to identify clinical correlates of extrapyramidal dysfunction in psychotic patients have focused predominantly on dyskinesia. For example, Gervin et al. (1998) pointed out that lower education and lower IQ were predisposing factors associated with dyskinesia in younger, never-treated patients with schizophrenia or schizophreniform disorder. In a more chronically ill but untreated patient sample, Fenton et al. (1994) found that low IQ and negative symptom severity were risk factors for dyskinesia. Moreover, in a subsequent paper, Fenton et al. (1997) further elaborated that dyskinesia and other movement disorders were more commonly found in individuals who met the criteria for a diagnosis of schizophrenia compared with those diagnosed with other forms of severe mental illness. Fenton and other recent authors (Fenton et al. 1994) have also suggested that in many patients with facial dyskinesia, who also present with intellectual impairment and negative symptoms, the motor abnormalities are part of the syndrome referred to historically as hebephrenia or deficit syndrome schizophrenia. This opinion echoed the earlier findings of Rogers (1985) and Turner (1989).

In an investigation of schizophrenic patients with and without evidence of abnormal involuntary movements, there were no differences in age, chronicity, education, or drug treatment that would distinguish the two groups (Manschreck et al. 1990). Yet patients with abnormal involuntary movements had greater evidence of voluntary motor abnormality; greater evidence of formal thought disorder, negative symptoms, and memory disturbance; and lower premorbid intellectual ability. This study is consistent with others (e.g., Fenton et al. 1994, 1997; Kopala et al. 1998; Waddington 1995) indicating complexity of abnormal involuntary motor features in schizophrenic disorder. The presence of these features suggests profound changes in cognition, lower likelihood of recovery, and greater severity of psychopathologic features. These observations also suggest that spontaneous or neuroleptic-related abnormal involuntary movements have a pathophysiology related to the syndrome of schizophrenia (Crow et al. 1983; Iager et al. 1986; Manschreck 1989).

Risk Factors and Mechanisms of Basal Ganglia Dysfunction

Studies of the prevalence and importance of basal ganglia dysfunction in schizophrenia have been compromised by medication side effects and a past perspective that considers schizophrenia separate from neurological disorders. Increasing numbers of studies of first-episode, never-medicated subjects, using rating scales that are sensitive to movement disorders, have established that basal ganglia dysfunction is surprisingly prevalent in these neuroleptic-naïve patients. Not only are abnormal involuntary movements observed, but parkinsonism is as well. The relationship of basal ganglia dysfunction to the course and prognosis of schizophrenia needs further investigation, particularly in the context of the availability of antipsychotic drugs with significantly reduced motor side effects.

Numerous investigators have examined the role of genetic factors and their relative contribution to the development of parkinsonism and dyskinesia. A review (Wolff and O'Driscoll 1999) of high-risk subjects and family members of probands with schizophrenia concluded that a relationship was present between genetic risk and abnormalities on neurological examination. However, few studies focused specifically on basal ganglia function. Compared with healthy subjects, signs of increased tone, tremor, or chorea have been found to be more common in relatives of patients with schizophrenia (Griffiths et al. 1998); however, signs of extrapyramidal disorder were not increased in siblings of patients with schizophrenia compared with healthy volunteers (Chen et al. 2000). Another study of schizophrenia "spectrum" conditions indicated increased dyskinesia, particularly in schizotypal subjects (Cassady et al. 1998), although mean scores for parkinsonism were not significantly increased. Interestingly, dyskinesia in the spectrum subjects was ameliorated by the second of two amphetamine challenges, whereas dyskinesia in healthy comparison subjects was increased after the first amphetamine challenge and persisted at a high level after the second. Spontaneous dyskinesia was related to the severity of positive symptoms, and amelioration of dyskinesia by amphetamine was related to the severity of negative symptoms. The latter finding suggests that dopaminergic mechanisms may well be involved in these motor disorders but in complex ways that likely depend on alterations in the balance of neurotransmitters on cortical-striatal-thalamic circuitry.

Other risk factors for abnormal basal ganglia function in first-episode patients prior to exposure to antipsychotic medication have received limited attention. Age, duration of symptoms prior to assessment, and age at onset of psychosis were reported to be unrelated to signs of basal ganglia dysfunction (Chatterjee et al. 1995); however, extrapyramidal symptoms and signs in never-medicated patients at first episode were related to a history of severe mental illness in the family and to poor premorbid functioning (Honer et al., in press).

Dissection of the circuitry related to basal ganglia dysfunction in schizophrenia may be significantly advanced by the application of functional imaging techniques. Although not yet applied to never-medicated subjects, functional magnetic resonance imaging techniques demonstrate that specific posterior regions within the basal ganglia fail to be activated by motor tasks in patients with schizophrenia (Menon et al. 2001). These same regions showed correlations in activity with the thalamus, suggesting impaired neurocircuitry.

Neurological Nonlocalizing ("Soft") Signs

The application of newer techniques of central nervous system (CNS) investigation, such as functional neuroimaging, has generated interest in finding meaningful connections between clinical observations and the underlying neuropathology of schizophrenia. A review of the literature on neurological signs (Heinrichs and Buchanan 1988) demonstrated a higher prevalence of such signs in schizophrenia than in nonpsychiatric and psychiatric control subjects, including some degree of temporal stability, a lack of medication effect (i.e., signs appear to be a stable trait), a trend toward increased neurological soft sign prevalence in males, and a modest influence of age and socioeconomic status. The majority of studies have found abnormalities in integrative sensory function, such as bilateral extinction, left–right confusion, impaired audiovisual integration, agraphesthesia, and astereognosis. Other areas frequently found to show difficulties include motor coordination (e.g., balance, station and gait, and general coordination) and motor sequencing (e.g., performance of complex sequences of action, such as repetitive alternations of hand position). These findings indicate that basic mechanisms of sensory input and motor output are not disturbed, but rather that higher-order functional integration of sensory and motor responses is impaired.

Associations between the occurrence of neurological signs and thought disorder and cognitive impairment (including performance on mental status examination) appear to be fairly robust. Similar associations have been identified for negative symptoms and chronicity of illness; moreover, first-degree biological relatives of schizophrenic probands appear to have increased evidence of neurological signs.

One major difficulty in interpreting the literature on this subject has been the application of various nonstandardized examination techniques. To remedy this, Buchanan and Heinrichs (1989) developed the Neurological Evaluation Scale (NES), a structured examination rating scale with respectable reliability. Since the Heinrichs and Buchanan review, efforts to investigate the significance of neurological signs have produced a number of interesting findings. For example, Gupta et al. (1995) found that 23% of neuroleptic-naïve and 46% of medicated schizophrenic subjects had evidence of neurological signs, whereas others (Chen et al. 2000; Ismail et al. 1998a) have found high prevalences of neurological abnormalities in schizophrenic patients and their siblings. Wong et al. (1997) found additionally that neurological signs are associated with negative symptoms, poor psychosocial performance, and increased cognitive impairment. Interestingly, Flashman et al. (1996) suggested that neurological signs are not indicative of global cognitive impairment, but rather are a manifestation of a localizable behavioral deficit of the neural systems subserving motor speed, coordination, and sequencing, suggesting a frontal subcortical circuit disturbance in schizophrenia.

Primitive Reflexes

There is some evidence that primitive reflexes (e.g., grasp and suck reflexes) as assessed in the NES may reflect cerebral dysfunction common in schizophrenia. Primitive reflexes are present in infants and children but gradually disappear as myelination takes place; however, these reflexes often occur in adults who suffer from brain disease. According to Youssef and Waddington (1988), it is significantly more common to find primitive reflexes in schizophrenic patients with abnormal involuntary movements than among those without involuntary movements, which led to the conclusion that patients with TD suffer from an excess of cerebral dysfunction. The most cautious statement that can be made with regard to the significance of primitive reflexes is that they probably have little or no diagnostic or localizing value because they are nonspecific, but they can be seen as a reflection of neurological dysfunction when they occur in adolescents and adults with schizophrenia (possibly due to disordered neurodevelopment).

Abnormalities in Handedness

Lateralization refers to the differential activation of left and right hemispheres for motor, perceptual, cognitive, and other functions. This implies a specific dominance or specialization for different brain tasks, such as language. In psychopathology, the possible relationship of lateralization to neurological and psychological features of schizophrenia has stimulated considerable interest.

One aspect of this focus has been on handedness in schizophrenia. The general finding, although not without exception, has been that there is excess left-handedness among schizophrenic subjects, suggesting altered lateralization (Boklage 1977). Because left-handedness is distributed normally in the population in the range of 7% to 10%, a higher prevalence suggests that lateralization has been modified, perhaps because of disease or CNS damage. In a related examination of this issue, Manschreck and Ames (1984) found a lack of consistency in lateralization (eye, hand, and foot preferences) in schizophrenia compared with control subjects, a phenomenon termed anomalous laterality. An anomalous laterality subject might, for example, be right-handed and right-eyed, but would kick with the left foot. Patients with anomalous laterality had greater motor, thought, and cognitive disturbances than schizophrenic subjects who were consistently lateralized. This finding suggests that laterality may have an important pathogenetic connection to motor abnormality and other disturbances in schizophrenia.

Manoach et al. (1988) found heightened formal thought disorder among left-handed compared with right-handed schizophrenic subjects, and Manschreck et al. (1996) found that left-handed schizophrenic subjects performed more poorly on context memory. This finding and that of the UK Child Development Study (Crow et al. 1996) suggest that low lateralization of performance is associated with a higher risk for adult schizophrenia, although this claim warrants further study.

The measurement of handedness itself as an index of lateralization often suffers from methodological problems (Satz and Green 1999). The evaluation of handedness as in, for example, the Annett Scale depends on preference rather than performance. That is, subjects are asked to provide preferences for specific actions such as writing, throwing a ball, opening a jar, or cutting with scissors. The result of such probes is an estimate of right-, left-, or mixed handedness, a discontinuous measure presumably related to cerebral lateralization (Green et al. 1989a). However, an evaluation of actual performance ability in such activities offers a more sensitive assessment and generates a continuous quantitative measure. The senior author and colleagues have developed a tool to measure such ability: the line drawing task.

The line drawing task is simple, places minimal demand on the understanding of instructions or on previously learned skills, and is designed to give an estimate of laterality based on performance differences between hands. Using such a measure in samples that include schizophrenic subjects has led to interesting findings. For example, schizophrenic subjects are considerably less lateralized than control subjects. This means that schizophrenic subjects draw lines of similar straightness with either hand regardless of their stated preference. Individuals with such low levels of lateralization are referred to as poorly lateralized. Schizophrenic subjects with poor lateralization have an earlier age of onset and more negative symptoms, mannerisms, and parkinsonian features than control subjects (Manschreck et al., in submission). This set of observations linking one aspect of brain function associated with hemispheric dominance to clinical features suggests a connection between deviant cerebral development and the occurrence of certain psychopathological features in schizophrenia. Specifically, poor lateralization, early onset, and both voluntary and involuntary motor abnormalities appear to be linked among some patients with schizophrenia.

Failures of Normal Neurological Maturation

In work designed to unravel the nature of neurological signs and the course of early-onset schizophrenia, Karp et al. (2001) evaluated neurological functioning in 21 adolescents with schizophrenia with onset of psychosis before age 13, compared with 27 matched (in age and sex) healthy comparison subjects. They found neurological signs at high frequency among the psychopathologic subjects, at rates comparable with those reported among adult schizophrenic subjects (Ismail et al. 1998b; Lane et al. 1996; Manschreck and Ames 1984). Distinguishing findings included lower IQ, sensory integration (face and hand) abnormalities, gaze impersistence, and corticospinal tract signs. A striking contrast was evidence of maturational loss of primitive reflexes, hypertonia, impaired coordination, and chorea with age among the healthy control subjects, a pattern not present among the childhood-onset cases. This demonstrates a failure of neurological maturation in the latter group. Other deviations from normal development in subjects with childhood onset of schizophrenia during adolescence include progressive loss of cortical and subcortical volume (Giedd et al. 1999) and decline in full-scale IQ (Bedwell et al. 1999).

In a related investigation of childhood-onset schizophrenia, premorbid speech and language impairments were associated with increased rates of three risk factors for schizophrenia: family history, familial eye tracking disturbance, and obstetrical complications (Nicolson et al. 2000).

Congenital Neurological Features (Minor Physical Anomalies)

Minor physical anomalies are modest deviations in physical characteristics that have been noted frequently in a variety of developmental disorders. They include such features as low-seated ears, curved fifth finger, high-steepled palate, partial syndactyly of the two middle toes, and malformed ears. These anomalies are believed to be indicators of ectodermal deviations that occur in the developing fetus. Because the CNS also derives from ectodermal tissue, the presence of excess physical anomalies is believed to be related to abnormal development of the CNS (Guy et al. 1983). Minor physical anomalies have been found in various conditions, including hyperactivity, autism, epilepsy, learning disabilities, and mental retardation (Lohr and Flynn 1993).

There is some evidence that abnormal prenatal development is associated with some cases of schizophrenia. Prenatal complications that may contribute to the occurrence of both physical anomalies and CNS deficits in schizophrenia include maternal disease or infection, dietary deficiency, hypoxia, rubella, bleeding, fetal distress, and toxemia (Guy et al. 1983). If schizophrenia has a neurodevelopmental source, then patients with the disorder should have an excess of minor physical anomalies. Studies of the prevalence of minor physical anomalies in schizophrenic patients compared with normal control subjects have found an excess of these anomalies in schizophrenia (Green et al. 1989b). Minor physical anomalies in schizophrenia are not limited to one body region but often include abnormalities of the feet as well as unusually large or small head circumference. Minor physical anomalies occur in other disorders but not with such high frequency as in schizophrenia, and this has suggested to some that there is a degree of specificity to schizophrenia among the psychotic disorders (Green et al. 1994). Siblings of schizophrenic patients do not appear to have an increase in minor physical anomalies, suggesting that the neural events reflected by such anomalies may be nongenetic in origin.

Eye Tracking Disturbances

Some of the most consistent neurological signs have to do with ocular movements. Among those reported by Stevens (1987) are absence and avoidance of eye contact, staring, changes in blink rate (often increased) and the glabellar reflex, pupillary inequality, and inability to converge. But the best studied of the ocular movement disturbances is eye tracking. In 1908, Diefendorf and Dodge (Levy et al. 1993) reported that some persons with schizophrenia exhibit eye movement abnormalities. The movements could be photographed and were detectable on careful neurological examination. During the 1970s Holzman and colleagues (Levy et al. 1993) extended the investigation of oculomotor function in schizophrenia. Using newer techniques of measurement, these investigators found that the oculomotor abnormalities or eye tracking disturbances were of two types. One disturbance affects smooth pursuit (matching the velocity of eye movement to the velocity of a moving target so as to stabilize the target's image on the retina). The other type affects saccades (which permit corrective speeding up or slowing down of eye movement to correspond to the target velocity more accurately). Schizophrenic patients demonstrate dysfunction primarily in smooth pursuit, but there is also an increased frequency of saccades based on this compensatory mechanism.

Studies indicate that 65% of schizophrenic patients and about 40% of their first-degree relatives show saccadic intrusions and failures in smooth pursuit movements. These abnormalities in eye movements are not explained by symptoms of the disorder, medication side effects, or other factors. They seem to be specific to schizophrenia, although not unique, since they occur in about 8% of normal subjects. Approximately 14% of mood-disordered patients show similar abnormalities.

Recent work has suggested that eye tracking disturbances may be characterized as a vulnerability marker for schizophrenia. Their occurrence in healthy, unaffected biological relatives tends to support this concept (Levy et al. 1993). Other investigators examining the deficit syndrome (composed of primary and enduring negative symptoms of psychopathology) have suggested that eye tracking disturbance may be associated with this possible subtype of schizophrenia (Ross 2000).

Cognitive Disturbances

In the past decade the study of recovery and outcome in schizophrenia has inspired a renewed emphasis on the cognitive dimension of the disorder (Harvey 2000). The reasons are several. First, cognitive impairment is widely prevalent and affects nearly every cognitive function (Harvey and Keefe 1997). Second, it is not the result of other symptoms or drug treatment; hence, it is a central component of the disorder. Third, not only is cognitive impairment present at the onset of diagnosable illness (i.e., at the appearance of psychosis), but various studies, including those of high-risk samples, indicate that it is present long before (Crow et al. 1996). Fourth, cognitive disturbance is the strongest predictor of overall outcome in schizophrenia (Harvey 1997). Fifth, cognitive impairments are largely responsible for the functional deficits that create much of the disability and indirect costs associated with schizophrenia (Harvey 2000). Finally, there are indications that the newer, second-generation antipsychotic medications, including clozapine, may improve cognitive performance (McGurk and Meltzer 2000).

However, despite the recognition that cognitive disturbance is a central feature, no cognitive deficit specific to schizophrenia has emerged from years of research. Rather, the picture is that of a range of deficits, affecting a variety of cognitive domains and suggesting a diffuse underlying neurophysiology and neuropathology. Efforts to connect specific deficits to functional consequences have been helpful in identifying promising targets for intervention, including medication strategies and rehabilitative efforts (Green 1996; Green and Braff 2001). The following features of cognitive dysfunction have been widely recognized and associated with schizophrenia.

Attention

Various elements of attention have been found deviant in schizophrenia. These include vigilance (or sustained attention), selective attention (including distractibility), and early visual processing (Oltmanns and Neale 1975). Vigilance performance has been shown to be related to functional outcome in schizophrenic patients (Green 1996). Measured with the continuous performance test, vigilance is the ability to discriminate targets from nontargets under various conditions for varied lengths of time, as in a radar operation task. Although selective attention has been identified as a commonly compromised feature of schizophrenic cognitive function, it appears to be responsive to medication and has not been identified as a key characteristic in functional success.

Memory

There are several types of memory disturbance in schizophrenia. The distinction between *explicit* memory (conscious recollection of prior events) and *implicit* memory (occurring outside of conscious awareness, as in improved performance resulting from a series of learning trials) has been useful (Squire 1992). Schizophrenic patients tend to show greater deficits in explicit memory in tasks such as recognition and recall of word lists, and to show relative intactness in implicit memory in ones such as motor skill tasks in which practice improves performance.

Working memory, which is similar in concept to short-term memory, refers to the ability to maintain memory representations temporarily, as in remembering a phone number. Verbal working memory (e.g., identifying and distinguishing recent auditory stimuli from other presented stimuli) and spatial working memory (e.g., remembering where in the lot a car is parked) have been distinguished, with the neuroanatomy of the latter mapped in primates. These studies indicate that neurons in prefrontal cortex appear to maintain a representation of the stimulus when the stimulus is no longer in the visual field. Schizophrenic subjects show deficits in spatial working memory compared with control subjects (Park and Holzman 1992).

Executive Functions

Executive functions include a range of abilities associated with organizing, planning, problem solving, and the initiation, maintenance, and shifting of responses to environmental demands. The Wisconsin Card Sorting Test

(WCST) has become the main measure of executive functioning in schizophrenia research (Palmer and Heaton 2000). This test involves matching a series of cards to one of four target cards on the basis of three forms of rule (color, shape, or number). Subjects are not told how to match the cards, but only whether their match is right or wrong; hence, they are to work out the proper rule. After a certain number of responses, the rules change. Schizophrenic subjects have problems performing this task. Considerable interest in the WCST has been generated by the demonstration that normal controls activate prefrontal cortex when performing this task, but schizophrenic patients do not (Weinberger et al. 1986). However, there is also evidence that cortical-subcortical connections are relevant to these functions as well (Cummings 1993). Deficits in executive functions (as well as vigilance and working memory) appear to be important for achieving various forms of social and functional outcome, and hence are seen as a significant component of the burden of this illness.

Formal Thought Disorder

Some patients with schizophrenia experience a range of difficulties in language function. These difficulties often depend on speech, attention, and memory mechanisms. Among the notable problems are derailment, poverty of content of speech, and associational disturbances. Schizophrenic speech is often highly repetitive, difficult to comprehend, and at times uninformative, and it may contain neologisms, oddities of expression, and illogical features. There is no clear aphasic disturbance in schizophrenia.

Formal thought disorder is the clinical term used to describe manifestations of language abnormalities in schizophrenia. Studies using clinical rating scales have found that 50% of patients with schizophrenia manifest some form of communication disorder at a moderate or greater level. The most common abnormalities are in the domains of verbal productivity (e.g., the amount of speech produced) and speech connectedness (e.g., the logic, coherence, and referential nature of speech). Much less common (less than 10%) are disorders such as neologisms and word approximations (Peralta et al. 1992). These disturbances are not diagnostic; rather, they are nonspecific features. However, there is some evidence for communication disorder being useful in distinguishing mood disorders (both bipolar and depressive disorders) from schizophrenia (Andreasen and Grove 1986; Cuesta and Peralta 1993). Poverty of speech is an indicator of risk for poor functional outcome; as alogia, it is considered a negative symptom. It is associated with reductions in emotional tone and in vocal inflection and spontaneity. Disconnected patterns of speech are associated with bizarre behavior and inappropriate affect.

Motor Disturbances

In addition to the range of movement abnormalities already discussed in this chapter, patients with schizophrenia have pronounced difficulties with motor speed and visual motor skills. The speed of reaction (reaction time) has long been observed to be disordered in schizophrenia. But even simpler responses, such as tapping speed and motor synchrony, are often disturbed as well (Manschreck et al. 1981). General clumsiness, problems with repetitive movements, and disruption of sequential motor actions add to the cognitive disturbance burden of the condition. Motor response (relevant to skill building), efficient reaction to new stimuli, and overall functional effectiveness are compromised as a result.

Awareness of Illness

Disturbed awareness of illness—impaired ability to recognize and understand symptoms and illness, or lack of insight—has been studied recently because it is highly prevalent and is associated with poor adherence to treatment and poor outcome; moreover, affected patients with severe awareness deficits may not reliably report their symptoms, thus impeding diagnostic and treatment processes. There have been a number of attempts to link this disturbance to possible cognitive underpinnings, but no definitive results as yet.

Conclusion

The concept that schizophrenia is a disease of the brain is well established; however, the complexity and subtle nature of this disorder have at times made it difficult to diagnose and to characterize. Its clinical heterogeneity creates enormous challenges to establishing firm, generalizable observations, and its probable etiological heterogeneity is a sober reminder of the limitations of our knowledge.

This chapter has dealt with the neurological comorbidity and features of schizophrenia. Comorbid diseases demonstrate the clinical importance of being aware of different brain disorders that mimic the presentation of and that complicate the course and management of schizophrenia. Despite claims that they are the result of treatment or other disorders, the neurological features that we consider now to be a part of schizophrenia remain only partly understood. The need to identify, measure, characterize, and fit these features into models of etiology, pathogenesis, and pathophysiology has become clearer. These features may well be a future source for laboratory diagnostic testing and clinical response monitoring.

Indeed, an important argument can be made that the care of patients with schizophrenia must involve some routine neuropsychological testing to determine the nature of cognitive deficits and thereby plan appropriate interventions. The extent and form of rehabilitative services for any individual demands an understanding of his or her cognitive functioning. Although extensive motor and neuropsychiatric assessments have often been limited to academic centers, the clinical importance of quantifying cognitive functions, given the strong association between schizophrenia, cognitive deficits, and functional outcome, cannot be overestimated. The results of IQ testing provide significant data on verbal and nonverbal abilities. Specific tests of motor skills (grooved pegboard), executive functioning (WCST), and verbal learning (Hopkins or California verbal learning tests) are also easily performed in routine clinical settings by a psychologist. Although schizophrenia is indeed a neurocognitive disorder, the referral for testing is unlikely to come from any medical provider other than the psychiatrist or community mental health center, because few other practitioners may be aware of the need to perform cognitive testing in these patients.

References

American Psychiatric Association: Diagnostic and Statistical Manual of Mental Disorders, 4th Edition, Text Revision. Washington, DC, American Psychiatric Association, 2000

Andreasen NC, Grove WM: Thought, language, and communication in schizophrenia: diagnosis and prognosis. Schizophr Bull 12:348–359, 1986

Arieti S: Volition and value: a study based on catatonic schizophrenia, in Moral Values and the Superego Concept in Psychoanalysis. Edited by Post SC. New York, International University Press, 1972, pp 275–288

Barnes TR: A rating scale for drug-induced akathisia. Br J Psychiatry 154:672–676, 1989

Bedwell JS, Keller B, Smith AK, et al: Why does postpsychotic IQ decline in childhood-onset schizophrenia? Am J Psychiatry 156:1996–1997, 1999

Berrios GE, Chen EYH: Recognizing psychiatric symptoms: relevance to the diagnostic process. Br J Psychiatry 163:308–314, 1993

Bleuler E: Dementia Praecox or the Group of Schizophrenias (1911). Translated by Zinkin J. New York, International Universities Press, 1950

Boklage CE: Schizophrenia, brain asymmetry development, twinning: cellular relationship with etiologic and possibly prognostic implications. Biol Psychiatry 12:19–35, 1977

Browne S, Clarke M, Gervin M, et al: Determinants of neurological dysfunction in first episode schizophrenia. Psychol Med 30:1433–1441, 2000

Buchanan RW, Heinrichs DW: The Neurological Evaluation Scale (NES): structured instrument for the assessment of neurological signs in schizophrenia. Psychiatry Res 27:335–350, 1989

Caligiuri MP, Lohr JB, Jeste DV: Parkinsonism in neuroleptic-naïve schizophrenic patients. Am J Psychiatry 150:1343–1348, 1993

Cassady SL, Adami H, Moran M, et al: Spontaneous dyskinesia in subjects with schizophrenia spectrum personality. Am J Psychiatry 155:70–75, 1998

Chambers RA, Krystal JH, Self DW: A neurobiological basis for substance abuse comorbidity in schizophrenia. Biol Psychiatry 50:71–83, 2001

Chatterjee A, Chakos M, Koreen A, et al: Prevalence and clinical correlates of extrapyramidal signs and spontaneous dyskinesia in never-medicated schizophrenic patients. Am J Psychiatry 152:1724–1729, 1995

Chen YLR, Chen YHE, Mak FL: Soft neurological signs in schizophrenia and character disorders. J Nerv Ment Dis 188:84–89, 2000

Chorfi M, Moussaoui D: Les schizophrènes jamais traités n'ont pas de mouvements anormaux type dyskinésie tardive. L'Encéphale 9:263–265, 1985

Crow TJ, Cross AJ, Johnstone EC, et al: Abnormal involuntary movements in schizophrenia: Are they related to the disease process or its treatment? Are they associated with changes in dopamine receptors? J Clin Psychopharmacol 2:336–340, 1982

Crow TJ, Owens DGC, Johnstone EC, et al: Does tardive dyskinesia exist? Mod Probl Pharmacopsychiatry 21:206–219, 1983

Crow TJ, Done DJ, Sacker A: Cerebral lateralization is delayed in children who later develop schizophrenia. Schizophr Res 22:181–185, 1996

Cuesta MJ, Peralta V: Does formal thought disorder differ among patients with schizophrenic, schizophreniform and manic schizoaffective disorders? Schizophr Res 10:151–158, 1993

Cummings JL: Frontal-subcortical circuits and human behavior. Arch Neurol 50:873–880, 1993

Degwitz R: Extrapyramidal motor disorders following long-term treatment with neuroleptic drugs, in Psychotropic Drugs and Dysfunctions of the Basal Ganglia. Edited by Crane GE, Gardner R Jr. Washington, DC, U.S. Public Health Service, 1969

Doody GA, Johnstone EC, Sanderson TL, et al: "Pfropfschizophrenie" revisited: schizophrenia in people with mild learning disability. Br J Psychiatry 173:145–153, 1998

Dretler J: Influence de l'encéphalite épidémique sur la schizophrénie. L'Encéphale 30:656–670, 1935

Duke PJ, Pantelis C, McPhillips MA, et al: Comorbid non-alcohol substance misuse among people with schizophrenia: epidemiological study in central London. Br J Psychiatry 179:509–513, 2001

Fahn S: Treatment of tardive dyskinesia, use of dopamine depleting drugs. Clin Neuropharmacol 6:151–158, 1983

Fenn DS, Moussaoui D, Hoffman WF, et al: Movements in never-medicated schizophrenics: a preliminary study. Psychopharmacology 123:206–210, 1996

Fenton WS: Prevalence of spontaneous dyskinesia in schizophrenia. J Clin Psychiatry 61 (suppl 4):10–14, 2000

Fenton WS, Wyatt RJ, McGlashan TH: Risk factors for spontaneous dyskinesia in schizophrenia. Arch Gen Psychiatry 51:643–650, 1994

Fenton WS, Blyler CR, Wyatt RJ, et al: Prevalence of spontaneous dyskinesia in schizophrenic and non-schizophrenic psychiatric inpatients. Br J Psychiatry 171:265–268, 1997

Flashman LA, Flaum M, Gupta S, et al: Soft signs and neuropsychological performance in schizophrenia. Am J Psychiatry 153:526–532, 1996

Gervin M, Browne S, Lane A, et al: Spontaneous abnormal involuntary movements in first-episode schizophrenia and schizophreniform disorder: baseline rate in a group of patients from an Irish catchment area. Am J Psychiatry 155:1202–1206, 1998

Giedd NJ, Jeffries NO, Blumenthal J, et al: Childhood-onset schizophrenia: progressive brain changes during adolescence. Biol Psychiatry 46:892–898, 1999

Green MF: What are the functional consequences of neurocognitive deficits in schizophrenia? Am J Psychiatry 153:321–330, 1996

Green MF, Braff DL: Translating the basic and clinical cognitive neuroscience of schizophrenia to drug development and clinical trials of antipsychotic medications. Biol Psychiatry 49:374–384, 2001

Green MF, Satz P, Smith C, et al: Is there atypical handedness in schizophrenia? J Abnorm Psychol 98:57–61, 1989a

Green MF, Satz P, Gaier DJ, et al: Minor physical anomalies in schizophrenia. Schizophr Bull 15:91–99, 1989b

Green MF, Satz P, Christenson C: Minor physical anomalies in schizophrenia patients, bipolar patients, and their siblings. Schizophr Bull 20:433–440, 1994

Griffiths TD, Sigmundsson T, Takei N, et al: Neurological abnormalities in familial and sporadic schizophrenia. Brain 121:191–203 1998

Gupta S, Andreasen C, Arndt S, et al: Neurological soft signs in neuroleptic-naïve and neuroleptic-treated schizophrenic patients and in normal comparison subjects. Am J Psychiatry 152:191–196, 1995

Guy JD, Majorski LV, Wallace CJ, et al: The incidence of minor physical anomalies in adult male schizophrenics. Schizophr Bull 9:571–582, 1983

Harvey P: Formal thought disorder in schizophrenia: characteristics and cognitive underpinnings, in Cognition in Schizophrenia. Edited by Sharma T, Harvey P. New York, Oxford University Press, 2000, pp 107–125

Harvey PD, Keefe RSE: Cognitive impairment in schizophrenia and implications of atypical neuroleptic treatment. CNS Spectr 2:41–55, 1997

Heinrichs DW, Buchanan RW: Significance and meaning of neurological signs in schizophrenia. Am J Psychiatry 145:11–18, 1988

Honer WG, Kopala L, Rabinowitz J: Prevalence and severity of movement disorders in first-episode, neuroleptic-exposed and non-exposed patients with psychosis. Schizophr Res (in press)

Hyde TM, Weinberger DR: Seizures and schizophrenia. Schizophr Bull 23:611–622, 1997

Iager AC, Kirch DG, Jeste DV, et al: Defect symptoms and abnormal involuntary movements in schizophrenia. Biol Psychiatry 21:751–755, 1986

Ismail BT, Cantor-Graae E, McNeil TF: Neurological abnormalities in schizophrenic patients and their siblings. Am J Psychiatry 155:84–89, 1998a

Ismail BT, Cantor-Graae E, Cardenal S, et al: Neurological abnormalities in schizophrenia: clinical, etiological and demographic correlates. Schizophr Res 30:229–238, 1998b

Kahlbaum K: Catatonia. [Die Katatonie oder das Spannungs-Irresein. Berlin, Hirschwald, 1874]. Translated by Levij Y, Priden T. Baltimore, MD, Johns Hopkins University Press, 1973

Karp BI, Garvey M, Jacobsen LK, et al: Abnormal neurologic maturation in adolescents with early onset schizophrenia. Am J Psychiatry 158:118–122, 2001

Klawans HL: Introduction: symposium on tardive dyskinesia. Clin Neuropharmacol 6:75, 1983

Kopala L, Good K, Fredrikson D, et al: Risperidone in first-episode schizophrenia: improvement in symptoms and pre-existing extrapyramidal signs. Int J Psychiatry Clin Pract 2 (suppl):S19–S25, 1998

Kraepelin E: Dementia Praecox and Paraphrenia. Edinburgh, E & S Livingstone, 1919

Lane A, Colgan K, Moynihan F, et al: Schizophrenia and neurological soft signs: gender differences in clinical correlates and antecedent factors. Psychiatry Res 64:105–114, 1996

Leucht S, Pitschel-Walz G, Kissling AD: Efficacy and extrapyramidal side-effects of the new antipsychotics olanzapine, quetiapine, risperidone, and sertindole compared to conventional antipsychotics and placebo: a meta-analysis of randomized controlled trials. Schizophr Res 35:51–68, 1999

Levy DL, Holzman PS, Matthysse S, et al: Eye-tracking dysfunction and schizophrenia: a critical perspective. Schizophr Bull 19:461–536, 1993

Lohr JB, Flynn K: Minor physical anomalies in schizophrenia and mood disorders. Schizophr Bull 19:551–556, 1993

Lund CE, Mortimer AM, Rogers D, et al: Motor, volitional and behavioral disorders in schizophrenia, I: assessment using the modified Rogers scale. Br J Psychiatry 158:323–327, 1991

Malaspina D, Goetz RR, Friedman JH, et al: Traumatic brain injury and schizophrenia in members of schizophrenia and bipolar disorder pedigrees. Am J Psychiatry 158:440–446, 2001

Manoach DS, Maher BA, Manschreck TC: Left handedness and thought disorder in the schizophrenias. J Abnorm Psychol 97:97–99, 1988

Manschreck TC: Motor abnormalities in schizophrenic disorders, in Handbook of Schizophrenia, Vol 1: The Neurology of Schizophrenia. Edited by Nasrallah H, Weinberger D. Amsterdam, Elsevier North-Holland, 1986, pp 65–96

Manschreck TC: Motor and cognitive disturbances in schizophrenic disorders, in Schizophrenia: Scientific Progress. Edited by Tamminga C, Schulz SC. New York, Oxford University Press, 1989, pp 372–380

Manschreck TC, Ames D: Neurological features and psychopathology in schizophrenic disorders. Biol Psychiatry 19:703–719, 1984

Manschreck TC, Maher BA, Ader D: Formal thought disorder, the type–token ratio and disturbed voluntary motor behavior in schizophrenia. Br J Psychiatry 139:7–15, 1981

Manschreck TC, Maher BA, Rucklos ME, et al: Disturbed voluntary motor activity in schizophrenic disorder. Psychol Med 12:73–84, 1982

Manschreck TC, Keuthen NJ, Schneyer NL, et al: Abnormal involuntary movements and chronic schizophrenic disorders. Biol Psychiatry 27:150–158, 1990

Manschreck TC, Maher BA, Redmond D, et al: Laterality, memory, and thought disorder in schizophrenia. Neuropsychiatry Neuropsychol Behav Neurol 9:1–7, 1996

McGurk SR, Meltzer HY: The role of cognition in vocational functioning in schizophrenia. Schizophr Res 45:175–184, 2000

Mendez MF, Grau R, Doss RC, et al: Schizophrenia in epilepsy: seizure and psychosis variables. Neurology 43: 1073–1077, 1993

Menon V, Anagnoson RT, Glover GH, et al: Function MRI evidence for disrupted basal ganglia function in schizophrenia. Am J Psychiatry 158:646–649, 2001

Nasrallah HA, Weinberger DR (eds): Handbook of Schizophrenia, Vol 1: The Neurology of Schizophrenia. Amsterdam, Elsevier North-Holland, 1986

Nicolson R, Lenane M, Singaracharlu S, et al: Premorbid speech and language impairments in childhood-onset schizophrenia: association with risk factors. Am J Psychiatry 157:794–800, 2000

O'Dwyer JM: Schizophrenia in people with intellectual disability: the role of pregnancy and birth complications. J Intellect Disabil Res 41:238–251, 1997

Oltmanns TF, Neale JM: Schizophrenic performance when distractors are present: attentional deficit or differential task difficulty? J Abnorm Psychol 84:205–209, 1975

Onuma T, Adachi N, Hisano T, et al: 10-year follow-up study of epilepsy with psychosis. Jpn J Psychiatry Neurol 45:360–361, 1991

Palmer BW, Heaton RK: Executive dysfunction in schizophrenia, in Cognition in Schizophrenia. Edited by Sharma T, Harvey P. New York, Oxford University Press, 2000, pp 51–72

Park S, Holzman PS: Schizophrenics show spatial working memory deficits. Arch Gen Psychiatry 49:975–982, 1992

Peralta V, Cuesta MJ, de Leon J: Formal thought disorder in schizophrenia: a factor analytic study. Compr Psychiatry 33:105–110, 1992

Peralta V, Cuesta MJ, Martinez-Larrea A, et al: Differentiating primary from secondary negative symptoms in schizophrenia: a study of neuroleptic-naïve patients before and after treatment. Am J Psychiatry 157:1461–1466, 2000

Puri BK, Barnes TRE, Chapman MJ, et al: Spontaneous dyskinesia in first episode schizophrenia. J Neurol Neurosurg Psychiatry 66:76–78, 1999

Regier DA, Farmer ME, Rae DS, et al: Comorbidity of mental disorders with alcohol and other drug abuse. JAMA 26:2511–2518, 1990

Rogers D: The motor disorders of severe psychiatric illness: a conflict of paradigms. Br J Psychiatry 147:221–232, 1985

Rogers D: Motor Disorder in Psychiatry. Chichester, England, Wiley, 1992

Rogers D, Karki C, Bartlett C, et al: The motor disorders of mental handicap: an overlap with the motor disorders of severe psychiatric illness. Br J Psychiatry 158:97–102, 1991

Ross DE: The deficit syndrome and eye tracking disorder may reflect a distinct subtype within the syndrome of schizophrenia. Schizophr Bull 26:855–866, 2000

Sachdev P: Schizophrenia-like psychosis and epilepsy: the status of the association. Am J Psychiatry 153:325–336, 1998

Sanderson TL, Best JJ, Doody GA, et al: Neuroanatomy of comorbid schizophrenia and learning disability: a controlled study. Lancet 354:1867–1871, 1999

Sanderson TL, Doody GA, Best J, et al: Correlations between clinical and historical variables, and cerebral structural variables in people with mild intellectual disability and schizophrenia. J Intellect Disabil Res 45:89–98, 2001

Satz P, Green MF: Atypical handedness in schizophrenia: some methodological and theoretical issues. Schizophr Bull 25:63–78, 1999

Simpson GM, Angus JW: A rating scale for extrapyramidal side effects. Acta Psychiatr Scand Suppl 212:11–19, 1970

Slater E, Beard AW, Glithero E: The schizophrenia-like psychoses of epilepsy. Br J Psychiatry 109:95–150, 1963

Squire LR: Declarative and nondeclarative memory: multiple brain systems supporting learning and memory. J Cogn Neurosci 4:232–243, 1992

Steck H: Les syndrômes extrapyramidaux dans les maladies mentales. Archives Suisses de Neurologie et Psychiatrie 19:195–233, 1926; 20:92–136, 1927

Stevens JR: Neurology and neuropathology of schizophrenia, in Schizophrenia as a Brain Disease. Edited by Hern FA, Nasrallah HA. New York, Oxford University Press, 1987, pp 112–147

Taber's Cyclopedic Medical Dictionary. Philadelphia, PA, FA Davis, 1981

Trimble M: The Psychoses of Epilepsy. New York, Raven, 1991

Turner TH: Schizophrenia and mental handicap: an historical review, with implications for further research. Psychol Med 19:301–314, 1989

Turner TH: A diagnostic analysis of the casebooks of Ticehurst House Asylum, 1845–1890. Psychol Med Monogr Suppl 21:1–70, 1992

Waddington JL: Psychopathological and cognitive correlates of tardive dyskinesia in schizophrenia and other disorders treated with neuroleptic drugs. Behavioral Neurology of Movement Disorders 65:211–229, 1995

Weinberger DR, Berman KF, Zec RF: Physiologic dysfunction of dorsolateral prefrontal cortex in schizophrenia. Arch Gen Psychiatry 43:114–124, 1986

Whitehorn D, Kopala L: The changing significance of neuromotor dysfunction in the treatment of early psychosis: extrapyramidal signs and symptoms (EPSS) and the second-generation antipsychotic agents (in submission)

Wolff A-L, O'Driscoll GA: Motor deficits and schizophrenia: the evidence from neuroleptic-naïve patients and populations at risk. J Psychiatry Neurosci 24:304–314, 1999

Wong AHC, Voruganti LNP, Heslegrave RJ, et al: Neurocognitive deficits and neurological signs in schizophrenia. Schizophr Res 23:139–146, 1997

Youssef HA, Waddington JL: Primitive (developmental) reflexes and diffuse cerebral dysfunction in schizophrenia and bipolar affective disorder: overrepresentation in patients with tardive dyskinesia. Biol Psychiatry 23:791–796, 1988

Chapter 11

Prolactin- and Endocrine-Related Disorders in Schizophrenia

Diana O. Perkins, M.D., M.P.H.

Introduction

Neuroendocrine abnormalities are common in patients with schizophrenia, contributing to the risk of a variety of medical complications, including gynecomastia, galactorrhea, menstrual irregularities, and impaired sexual function. Although there is a lack of systematic data, other potential serious medical complications of neuroendocrine abnormalities, including breast cancer, osteoporosis, and prostate disorders, are of theoretical concern. In this chapter the effects of antipsychotics on neuroendocrine function are reviewed, with an emphasis on prolactin and its biological effects.

Antipsychotic Effects on Neuroendocrine Function

There are four major dopaminergic tracts in the central nervous system that may be affected by the dopaminergic antagonist activity of antipsychotics.

Dopamine antagonism of the mesolimbic tract is thought to result in reduction of positive symptoms, whereas dopamine antagonism of the me-
socortical track is thought to result in worsening of negative symptoms.
Dopaminergic antagonism of the nigrostriatal tract results in extrapyramidal symptoms, notably a parkinsonian syndrome. Most relevant to this
discussion is the fact that dopamine antagonism of the tuberoinfundibular
tract affects the function of the hypothalamic-pituitary-gonadal axis. The
pituitary gland is under inhibitory influence by dopaminergic neurons, so
antagonism of pituitary dopamine receptors releases the pituitary gland
from this inhibitory control, resulting in increased secretion of prolactin.

The Function of Prolactin

The clinical relevance of chronic high prolactin levels is not yet fully understood. Although one biological function of prolactin is to stimulate
mammary tissue to produce milk, over 300 other biological activities for
prolactin have been identified (Goffin et al. 2002). Prolactin is involved in
the regulation of reproductive function, for example, by inhibiting production of estrogen and testosterone by other tissues. Prolactin is also involved
in various homeostatic processes, including enhancement of immune system function (Neidhart 1998; Yu-Lee 2002), regulating angiogenesis (Corbacho et al. 2002), and osmoregulation (Shennan 1994).

Further research will likely reveal other roles for prolactin, because prolactin is produced by multiple tissues and interacts with multiple other
neurotransmitter, peptide, and hormonal systems. In addition to the anterior pituitary gland, numerous other brain areas produce prolactin, as do
breast tissue, placenta, uterus, prostate, and lymphocytes (Bole-Feysot et
al. 1998; Goffin et al. 2002). Other peptides are known to be affected by
or to affect prolactin levels; examples include estrogen, testosterone, leptin, galanin, somatostatin, calcitonin, bombesin-like peptides, neurotensin,
endothelins, neuropeptide Y, and cholecystokinin. In addition, neurotransmitter systems other than dopamine are affected by and/or affect
prolactin, including glutamate, aspartate, glycine, gamma-aminobutyric
acid (GABA), and nitric oxide. Although prolactin's role in reproductive
function is relatively well understood, prolactin's other homeostatic functions are less understood; nevertheless, the importance of prolactin is suggested by its widespread distribution and interaction with multiple other
systems.

In addition to pregnancy and lactation, many other factors affect serum
prolactin levels. A circadian variation exists in which levels increase substantially after the noontime meal, making fasting determinations more re-

liable than those obtained later in the day. In women, prolactin levels vary with time of menstrual cycle, with the peak at day 12 of the cycle and the nadir during the follicular phase. In addition, the number of live births plays a role in premenopausal women, with prolactin levels varying inversely with parity. In premenopausal women, high intake of saturated fats is associated with elevated prolactin levels (Wang et al. 1992; Wennbo and Tornell 2000). Primary hypothyroidism can also cause hyperprolactinemia, but values seldom exceed 50 ng/mL. The upper limit of normal prolactin levels is 23–25 ng/mL in women (obtained at day 3 of the cycle in premenopausal women) and 20 ng/mL in men.

Antipsychotic-Induced Hyperprolactinemia

Individuals with schizophrenia who are not taking antipsychotics do not appear to have elevated prolactin levels (Kuruvilla et al. 1992). Drugs with dopamine antagonist effects may result in prolactin elevation, and it is clear that the magnitude of hyperprolactinemia varies among the available antipsychotic medications, generally in proportion to the potency of D_2 antagonism. Prolactin elevation is greatest during treatment with typical antipsychotics and the atypical antipsychotic risperidone (Caracci and Ananthamoorthay 1999; David et al. 2000; Kleinberg et al. 1999); the atypical antipsychotics quetiapine (Hamner et al. 1996), clozapine (Kane et al. 1981), and ziprasidone (Goff et al. 1998) are not associated with prolactin elevation. With olanzapine, transient modest elevations of prolactin occur with initial treatment, but prolactin levels appear to normalize after a few weeks and remain normal with chronic treatment (Crawford et al. 1997).

Special populations may be especially vulnerable to antipsychotic-induced hyperprolactinemia. Women are clearly more sensitive than men to the effects of antipsychotics on prolactin (Crawford et al. 1997; David et al. 2000; Kleinberg et al. 1999). In a 6-week study, 63% of haloperidol-treated men compared with 98% of haloperidol-treated women had a prolactin level above the upper limit of normal (Crawford et al. 1997). In addition, children and adolescents may be especially sensitive to the prolactin-elevating effects of antipsychotics. In one study 100% (10/10) of haloperidol-treated, 70% (7/10) of olanzapine-treated, but no (0/15) clozapine-treated children (mean age 14, range 9–19 years) had elevated prolactin (Wudarsky et al. 1999). Olanzapine levels correlated with prolactin levels, and one olanzapine-treated girl with a prolactin level above 90 ng/mL experienced treatment-emergent galactorrhea (Alfaro et al. 2002).

The most prominent theory for explaining differences in prolactin elevation with atypical antipsychotics relates to the variable ability of antipsychotics to cross the blood–brain barrier (Kapur et al. 2002). The pituitary gland sits outside the blood–brain barrier and is exposed to peripheral blood; the rest of the brain is protected by the blood–brain barrier. Higher peripheral blood levels of a drug are needed to achieve adequate central nervous system levels if the drug does not readily cross the blood–brain barrier. Thus, the pituitary gland is exposed to higher levels of antipsychotics that do not readily cross the blood–brain barrier than the rest of the brain. This theory is supported by the results of an animal study that found relatively high pituitary-to-striatal dopamine receptor binding ratios for risperidone compared with quetiapine and olanzapine, with prolactin elevation highly correlated to this ratio (Kapur et al. 2002). In addition, the finding that prolactin is transiently elevated for 2–4 hours following administration of atypical antipsychotics (Turrone et al. 2002) is consistent with this theory. Other theories proposed to explain the lower risk of extrapyramidal side effects, including high ratios of affinity for serotonin (5-HT_2) to dopamine (D_2) antagonism (Meltzer 1989) and "loose" dopamine receptor binding (Kapur and Seeman 2001), do not readily explain differences in the prolactin-elevating properties of antipsychotics.

Clinical Implications of Hyperprolactinemia

The clinical consequences of high prolactin may be due either to the direct effects of prolactin on end organ tissues or to indirect effects, most obviously prolactin's regulation of other sex hormones, especially estrogen and testosterone. Prolactin's effects on the hypothalamus lead to decreased synthesis and release of estrogen and testosterone, so individuals with hyperprolactinemia may have secondary hypoestrogenemia and hypotestosteronemia.

Much of what is known about the clinical effects of hyperprolactinemia comes from studies of pituitary disease, such as prolactin-secreting tumors. The effects described in patients with prolactinoma may not be as common or may not be found in patients with antipsychotic-induced hyperprolactinemia, especially because the elevations in prolactin seen with prolactinoma tend to be markedly higher than those induced by antipsychotic medication. In addition, men and women have different risks of specific side effects related to hyperprolactinemia.

The following discussion describes studies of the clinical effects of antipsychotic-induced hyperprolactinemia, as well as studies of the clinical effects of high prolactin levels due to other causes. Unfortunately, most potential endocrine-related side effects of antipsychotics have not been well studied. There are some data regarding the risk of acute effects related to antipsychotic-induced hyperprolactinemia; however, little is known about the long-term side effects. In addition, because many studies rely on spontaneous reporting of sexual side effects, it is likely they underreport the frequency of sexual side effects because patients may be reluctant to volunteer this information without direct questioning (Hellewell 1998). For example, in one naturalistic study of galactorrhea incidence in women treated with typical antipsychotics, 20 of 28 women who developed galactorrhea failed to spontaneously report this side effect on general inquiry by the treating physician about medication side effects (Windgassen et al. 1996).

Breast

Prolactin normally stimulates breast tissue growth, differentiation, and lactation. Gynecomastia (breast enlargement) and galactorrhea (lactation) are expected consequences of antipsychotic-induced hyperprolactinemia in both men and women, although the actual risk of breast-related side effects is not well delineated (Schreiber and Segman 1997). Estimates of the frequency of galactorrhea in women treated with typical antipsychotics vary, with reports of up to half of premenopausal women experiencing galactorrhea, but this side effect is rarely reported in men (Ghadirian et al. 1982; Gitlin 1994; Inoue et al. 1980; Windgassen et al. 1966). One of the few studies to date that has systematically inquired about breast changes naturalistically followed 150 women with schizophrenia treated for 75 days with a variety of typical antipsychotics (Windgassen et al. 1996). Nineteen percent (28/150) of the women admitted to galactorrhea. The mean prolactin value for these patients was 55 ng/mL, but 4 patients with galactorrhea had prolactin levels within the normal range. Previous pregnancy, premenopausal status, and neuroleptic dose were significantly associated with likelihood of galactorrhea. A meta-analysis of pivotal clinical trials comparing risperidone with placebo and/or haloperidol found that only 1.5% (7/451) of risperidone-treated and 3.3% (1/30) of haloperidol-treated women spontaneously reported galactorrhea (Kleinberg et al. 1999). No men in this study (n=1,330) spontaneously reported galactorrhea, and 0.5% (4/1032) of risperidone-treated men spontaneously reported gynecomastia. Because this study relied on spontaneous report, it is likely that these numbers greatly underestimate the true incidence of breast changes associated with risperidone and haloperidol.

Prolactin is thought by some to be a "promoter" of breast cancer, stimulating the growth of mammary tumor cells and potentially affecting the rate of progression of breast cancer (Goffin et al. 1999; Llovera et al. 2000). Theoretically, the risk of breast cancer would increase only with long-term high prolactin levels (Hankinson et al. 1999). The relationship of prolactin to breast cancer risk in postmenopausal women has been investigated in several studies, with some finding positive associations (Ingram et al. 1990; Rose and Pruitt 1981) and others finding no relationship (Bernstein et al. 1990; Secreto et al. 1983). The best study conducted to date is a large, well-designed, retrospective-prospective study examining premorbid prolactin levels with later risk of breast cancer conducted as part of the prospective Nurses' Health Study (Hankinson et al. 1999). In this study there was a doubling of breast cancer risk in women with prolactin levels greater than 14 ng/mL compared with those with prolactin levels less than 6.5 ng/mL. It is important to note that the investigators controlled for estrogen use (which could elevate prolactin and thus confound the study results) as well as other factors known to affect breast cancer risk. This magnitude of risk increase is similar to that found for estrogen replacement therapy (Writing Group for the Women's Health Initiative Investigators 2002).

Studies of breast cancer risk associated with drug-related prolactin elevations are at this point inadequate to permit any conclusions to be drawn. Methodological problems include the small number of women in most studies, and the duration of exposure to the prolactin-elevating drug may not be documented or may be of insufficient duration to influence risk. One study found the 5-year incidence of breast cancer in older (>50 years) chronically hospitalized women to be about 3/100, which is about 10-fold higher than the 5-year general population risk (Halbreich et al. 1996); however, most studies of chronic exposure to phenothiazines or haloperidol in chronically hospitalized patients do not find elevated risk of breast cancer (Costa et al. 1981; Goode et al. 1981; Mortensen 1987, 1994). The results of studies examining breast cancer risk with use of reserpine (an antihypertensive agent with prolactin elevation as a side effect) are mixed as well, with some studies finding elevated risk of breast cancer (Armstrong et al. 1976; Heinonen et al. 1974; Stanford et al. 1986) but others finding no relationship (Aromaa et al. 1976; Curb et al. 1982; Labarthe and O'Fallon 1980; Laska et al. 1975; Mack et al. 1975; Shapiro et al. 1984). These studies varied in the duration of exposure to reserpine, further complicating the interpretation of these results, because only long-term exposure to higher prolactin levels is theorized to influence breast cancer risk (Hankinson et al. 1999).

Thus the impact of antipsychotic-induced increases in prolactin on breast cancer risk is at this point theoretical at best, with no consistent data suggesting increased risk of breast cancer associated with long-term exposure to prolactin-elevating antipsychotics. However, the results from the prospective Nurses' Health Study (Hankinson et al. 1999) indicate that further study is needed.

Prostate and Testes

Prolactin normally stimulates cell growth in the prostate gland (probably through direct as well as through androgen-mediated mechanisms), although it is unclear what impact hyperprolactinemia may have on the prostate gland in humans. In animal studies high prolactin results in prostate gland inflammation and abnormal cell growth (Reiter et al. 1999). In men benign prostatic hypertrophy is associated with increased prolactin in some but not all studies (Saroff et al. 1980). Prolactin levels normally increase with age, potentially confounding the results of these studies. Prolactin levels may be increased in men with prostate cancer, but the prostate itself may produce prolactin, making cause and effect difficult to determine (Goffin et al. 2002; Harper et al. 1976). One case-control study found no increased risk of prostate cancer in antipsychotic-treated patients (Mortensen 1992), but there are no studies of risk of prostate cancer in patients with sustained antipsychotic-induced hyperprolactinemia.

Prolactin inhibits hypothalamic release of gonadotropin-releasing hormone (GRH), which in turn stimulates the pituitary to release luteinizing hormone (LH) and follicle-stimulating hormone (FSH), both of which regulate testicular function, including normal production of testosterone, and spermatogenesis. In other disease states, high prolactin levels are associated with decreased testosterone and decreased sperm production (Winters and Troen 1984). However, usual doses of antipsychotics do not appear to be associated with changes in LH, FSH, or testosterone in men with schizophrenia (Kaneda and Fujii 2000; Markianos et al. 1999; Siris et al. 1980; Smith et al. 2002), although in one study very high doses of haloperidol (30–60 mg/day) were associated with low testosterone levels (Rinieris et al. 1989). Because men are less sensitive to the prolactin-elevating effects of antipsychotic medications, there may be a risk for hypogonadism only with higher doses of prolactin-elevating antipsychotics. Longitudinal, prospective studies are needed before the impact of prolactin-elevating antipsychotics on the hypothalamic-pituitary-gonadal axis in men is understood.

Ovaries

The release of LH and FSH regulates ovarian function, including normal ovarian estrogen production. By inhibiting the hypothalamic release of GRH, high prolactin levels can lead to disrupted reproductive function, including irregular menses, amenorrhea, and a chronic low estrogen state.

Prevalence of irregular menses or amenorrhea is high (30%–78%) in women treated with typical antipsychotics (Beaumont et al. 1974; Ghadirian et al. 1982; Gingell et al. 1993; Sandison et al. 1960). Fewer systematically collected data are available for patients treated with the atypical antipsychotic risperidone, although there are numerous case reports of menstrual irregularities with risperidone treatment (Dickson et al. 1995; Kim et al. 1999, 2002) and several case reports of resolution of irregular menses after a switch from typical antipsychotics or risperidone to another atypical antipsychotic (Canuso et al. 1998; Dickson et al. 1995; Gazzola and Opler 1998).

Despite the common occurrence of amenorrhea associated with typical antipsychotics and risperidone, few studies have examined the impact of high prolactin on estrogen or testosterone directly, or the clinical impact of a low estrogen state related to antipsychotic medication. First, prolactin level per se has not been associated with likelihood of irregular menses (Kleinberg et al. 1999; Magharious et al. 1998). Only one study has found low estrogen levels to be associated with antipsychotic-induced hyperprolactinemia (Smith et al. 2002), with two studies finding no association between prolactin and estrogen (Canuso et al. 2002; Huber et al. 2001). In one of these studies two patients with very high prolactin levels (>100 ng/mL) did have very low estrogen, suggesting a threshold level of hyperprolactinemia that must be exceeded before a low estrogen state develops.

Menstrual cycle irregularities are associated with schizophrenia, even in women with schizophrenia who have never been treated with antipsychotic medications (Shader et al. 1970). Thus, the extent to which menstrual irregularities are due to some shared risk factor with schizophrenia, or are a secondary consequence of schizophrenia independent of antipsychotic treatment effects, is unclear. Case studies reporting improvement in menstrual function with reduction of prolactin, because of either a switch in antipsychotic (Canuso et al. 1998; Dickson et al. 1995; Gazzola and Opler 1998) or reduction in prolactin from the addition of a dopamine agonist (Beaumont et al. 1975; Correa et al. 1981; Siever 1981), suggest that antipsychotic-induced hyperprolactinemia may contribute to risk of menstrual irregularities. Further research is clearly needed, given the potential clinical importance of a chronic low estrogen state on cardiovascular health and risk of osteoporosis (Grady et al. 1992).

Osteoporosis

Both male and female patients with schizophrenia have a high prevalence of osteoporosis (Halbreich et al. 1995; Halbreich and Palter 1996; Keeley et al. 1997). In one study, bone density in patients with schizophrenia receiving typical antipsychotic drugs was reduced an average of 14% compared with healthy individuals (Baastrup et al. 1980).

Several mechanisms may contribute to risk of osteoporosis in individuals with schizophrenia, including direct affects of hyperprolactinemia, effects of chronic low estrogen or testosterone, and other lifestyle factors that are associated with both schizophrenia and risk of osteoporosis, including smoking, alcohol use, poor diet, lack of sun exposure, and polydipsia (Halbreich and Palter 1996). Prolactin affects vitamin D synthesis and intestinal absorption of calcium, and thus hyperprolactinemia may directly affect bone mineralization. Whether due to antipsychotic-induced hyperprolactinemia, some unknown factor related to schizophrenia, or a combination of these factors, a low estrogen state is clearly associated with increased risk of osteoporosis (Klibanski et al. 1988). As discussed earlier, the frequent finding of menstrual abnormalities and more recent studies examining estrogen levels in women with schizophrenia indicate that women with schizophrenia may be at increased risk for low estrogen levels. In a recent study, 62% (11/16) of women treated with a variety of antipsychotics had peak cycle estrogen levels below the lower limit of normal (Canuso et al. 2002). Several other studies have also reported low mean estrogen levels in women with schizophrenia compared with women without schizophrenia (Huber et al. 2001; Smith et al. 2002). Hypogonadism in men also increases risk of osteoporosis (Greenspan 1986); however, low testosterone level does not appear to be a common complication of antipsychotic treatment (Kaneda and Fujii 2000; Markianos et al. 1999; Siris et al. 1980).

Osteoporosis is associated with significant morbidity and mortality, and the clinical observation of increased risk of osteopenia and osteoporosis in patients with schizophrenia is clearly of concern. It is unclear if the chronic moderate hyperprolactinemia associated with some antipsychotics contributes to bone density loss in men or women with schizophrenia. Prospective data in women with hyperprolactinemia secondary to prolactinoma indicate that bone density loss correlates strongly with the extent of time spent amenorrheic, but poorly with the serum prolactin level (Biller et al. 1992). Further study is needed to more fully understand the actual risk to patients exposed to antipsychotics and to determine the relative contribution of potential contributory factors.

Sexual Function

The regulation of sexual function involves multiple brain regions, neurotransmitters, and hormones, and thus is complex (Meston and Frohlich 2000). Sexual interest or sexual function may be impaired directly because of schizophrenia (e.g., negative symptoms may include decreased interest generally, including interest in sex, and severe positive symptoms or social dysfunction may interfere with the ability to develop sexual relationships). Sexual interest or function may thus improve with antipsychotic treatment, or may be impaired as a side effect of antipsychotic treatment. For example, in a study of men with schizophrenia who were in stable relationships (51 taking antipsychotics, 20 drug free, and 51 healthy control subjects), untreated men reported the lowest levels of sexual desire or interest, with antipsychotic-treated men reporting greater interest than untreated men (but less than healthy controls) but decreased ability to maintain an erection and impaired orgasm, and decreased satisfaction with sexual performance (Aizenberg et al. 1995).

Unfortunately, there are few systematic data available regarding the frequency of impaired sexual interest or function with antipsychotic treatment, and almost all studies are cross-sectional. These studies find that 35%–60% of men treated with typical antipsychotics report erectile dysfunction (Aizenberg et al. 1995; Ghadirian et al. 1982; Kotin et al. 1976; Seagraves 1989). One study comparing sexual side effects in 41 haloperidol-treated and 75 clozapine-treated patients with schizophrenia found that similar proportions treated with either antipsychotic reported erectile or ejaculatory dysfunction (21%–27%) and decreased sexual desire (28%–33% of women and 57%–63% of men) during the initial 6 weeks of treatment (Hummer et al. 1999); however, only in the clozapine cohort did the proportion reporting impaired sexual desire significantly decrease with long-term treatment (for men, from an initial 53% at the beginning of treatment to 22% by week 18; for women, from an initial 23% to 0% by week 18). One other study examining sexual function in women treated with typical antipsychotics found a similar proportion (22%) reporting decreased ability to achieve orgasm with antipsychotic treatment (Ghadirian et al. 1982).

Antipsychotic medications theoretically may affect sexual interest and sexual response through multiple mechanisms. It is important to remember that antipsychotics affect multiple neurotransmitter systems that are involved in the sexual response, including (but not limited to) dopamine and serotonin (Meston and Frohlich 2000). High prolactin may directly impair libido, for example, through interaction with prolactin receptors in the hypothalamus. Prolactin may indirectly affect sexual interest and function through inhibition of estrogen and testosterone synthesis, because both of these hormones affect sexual interest and function in men and women. In addition, there is evidence from one study that hyperprolactinemia in childhood and adolescence (secondary to pituitary tumors) may be associated with very low interest in sex in early adulthood (Siimes et al. 1993).

Clinical Implications

Evaluation

Inquiry about potential endocrine-related symptoms should be routine when antipsychotic medications are prescribed. Monitoring should include changes in breast size, lactation, sexual interest and function, and, in women, menstrual history. Essential topics for discussion with patients include the subjective distress related to the emergence of any medication side effect and the impact of treatment-emergent side effects on willingness to take the antipsychotic medication. Patients will vary considerably in their subjective distress to sexual side effects (Wesselmann and Windgassen 1995), although the development of any sexual side effects is associated with increased risk of medication nonadherence (Perkins 2002). Long-term treatment adherence may benefit from education and discussion of the short- and long-term potential risks of hyperprolactinemia, and the risks and benefits of treatment (Hummer et al. 1999).

Prolactin levels should be addressed in patients who report clinical symptoms that potentially may be due to hyperprolactinemia, especially if risperidone, typical antipsychotics, or high doses of olanzapine are used. Women who report disturbances in menstrual function, especially premenopausal women who report amenorrhea, should be referred for further relevant medical evaluation, such as gynecological examination, pregnancy test, progesterone challenge test, or other appropriate studies to evaluate gonadal function and estrogen status. Although the relationship between antipsychotic treatment, hyperprolactinemia, and hypoestrogenemia is not yet established, women with chronic amenorrhea are at increased risk of hypoestrogenemia with resultant osteoporosis. Thus, a bone density scan should be considered in premenopausal women reporting long-standing amenorrhea. Finally, individuals with very high prolactin levels should be evaluated for a primary disorder of the pituitary or other medical cause.

Treatment

Although there are several theoretical concerns regarding antipsychotic-induced hyperprolactinemia, there is a lack of empiric evidence to guide clinicians. It is unclear whether asymptomatic hyperprolactinemia is of any clinical consequence, especially if the prolactin level is not extraordinarily elevated. In symptomatic patients with high prolactin levels, antipsychotic dose reduction should always be considered as a first option, because hyperprolactinemia is usually dose related. In addition, there are now several prolactin-sparing antipsychotics available, including quetiapine, olanzapine, and ziprasidone. Switching to one of these antipsychotics is thus a potential treatment option when dose reduction is not effective or feasible. Direct treatment of symptomatic hyperprolactinemia with a dopamine agonist (e.g., cabergoline, bromocriptine, amantadine) may be considered for patients who have had a good response to the current prolactin-elevating antipsychotic, who require depot antipsychotics, or who do not wish to switch medications (American Psychiatric Association 1997). There are numerous case reports of reduction of prolactin levels and resolution of prolactin-related side effects with bromocriptine (Beaumont et al. 1975) or amantadine (Correa et al. 1981; Siever 1981; Valevski et al. 1998) treatment. The major risk associated with dopamine agonist treatment is exacerbation of psychosis; therefore, patients should be monitored closely when dopamine agonists are first used. Finally, there is one published case report of sildenafil citrate improving sexual interest and sexual function in antipsychotic-treated patients with schizophrenia (Benatov et al. 1999). Further study is needed before sildenafil is routinely used to treat sexual dysfunction in patients with schizophrenia.

Although there is no clear evidence that antipsychotic-induced hyperprolactinemia affects breast cancer or prostate cancer risk, it seems prudent for physicians prescribing antipsychotics to patients with existing breast or prostate cancer to confer with the treating oncologist over choice of antipsychotic drug, and to avoid prolactin-elevating antipsychotics in this special population. In addition, until more data are available, for women with a significant family history of breast cancer it may be prudent to specifically mention the theoretical role of prolactin as a promoter of breast cancer when discussing selection of antipsychotic medication.

Finally, given the sensitivity of children and adolescents to the prolactin-elevating effects of antipsychotics, and the lack of systematic study of hyperprolactinemia on normal sexual maturation, a conservative approach to the treatment of adolescents with prolactin-elevating antipsychotics may be warranted. Although in adults the direct effects of hyperprolactinemia appear to be reversible, it is unknown whether this is the case during puberty.

Conclusion

Both the short-term and chronic medical consequences of hyperprolactinemia and related hypogonadism are of clear clinical concern. Confusing the clinical approach to these issues is the fact that the correlation between serum prolactin and sexual dysfunction in particular is not high. Thus, routine screening for potential prolactin-related side effects by direct inquiry should be performed prior to the institution of antipsychotic therapy and should be followed with routine direct questioning during treatment to elicit sexual side effects, which may not be reported either spontaneously or from general queries about side effects. Because patients may suffer sexual side effects with normal prolactin levels, and some with elevated prolactin levels remain asymptomatic, the clinical responses to follow-up questions will be more useful in dictating treatment than the measurement of prolactin levels without consideration of the clinical picture. Although asymptomatic hyperprolactinemia may often not be of clinical concern, persistent amenorrhea, regardless of the serum prolactin level, should be addressed to prevent bone density loss. It is to be hoped that future clinical research will further our understanding of the risk of serious medical consequences and medical management of hypothalamic-pituitary-gonadal alterations in patients with schizophrenia.

References

Aizenberg D, Zemishlany Z, Dorfman-Etrog P, et al: Sexual dysfunction in male schizophrenic patients. J Clin Psychiatry 5:137–141, 1995

Alfaro CL, Wudarsky M, Nicolson R, et al: Correlation of antipsychotic and prolactin concentrations in children and adolescents acutely treated with haloperidol, clozapine, or olanzapine. J Child Adolesc Psychopharmacol 12:83–91, 2002

American Psychiatric Association: Practice guidelines for the treatment of patients with schizophrenia. Am J Psychiatry 154 (suppl 4):1–62, 1997

Armstrong B, Skegg D, White G, et al: Rauwolfia derivatives and breast cancer in hypertensive women. Lancet 2:8–12, 1976

Aromaa A, Hakama M, Hakulinen T, et al: Breast cancer and use of rauwolfia and other antihypertensive agents in hypertensive patients: a nationwide case-control study in Finland. Int J Cancer 18:727–738, 1976

Baastrup P, Christiansen C, Transobol I: Calcium metabolism in schizophrenic patients on long-term neuroleptic therapy. Neuropsychobiology 6:56–59, 1980

Beaumont PJV, Gelder MG, Freissen HG, et al: The effects of phenothiazine on endocrine function: patients with inappropriate lactation and amenorrhoea. Br J Psychiatry 124:413–419, 1974

Beaumont P, Bruwer J, Pimstone B: Bromo-ergocryptine in the treatment of phenothiazine induced galactorrhea. Br J Psychiatry 126:285–288, 1975

Benatov R, Reznik I, Zemishlany Z: Sildenafil citrate (Viagra) treatment of sexual dysfunction in a schizophrenic patient. Eur Psychiatry 14:353–355, 1999

Bernstein L, Ross RK, Pike MC, et al: Hormone levels in older women: a study of post-menopausal breast cancer patients and healthy controls. Br J Cancer 61:298–302, 1990

Biller BM, Baum HB, Rosenthal DI, et al: Progressive trabecular osteopenia in women with hyperprolactinemic amenorrhea. J Clin Endocrinol Metab 75:692–697, 1992

Bole-Feysot C, Goffin V, Edery M, et al: Prolactin and its receptor: actions, signal transduction pathways, and phenotypes observed in prolactin receptor knockout mice. Endocr Rev 19:225–268, 1998

Canuso CM, Hanau M, Jhamb KK, et al: Olanzapine use in women with antipsychotic-induced hyperprolactinemia (letter). Am J Psychiatry 155:1458, 1998

Canuso CM, Goldstein JM, Wojcik J, et al: Antipsychotic medication, prolactin elevation, and ovarian function in women with schizophrenia and schizoaffective disorder. Psychiatry Res 111:11–20, 2002

Caracci G, Ananthamoorthay R: Prolactin levels in premenopausal women treated with risperidone compared with those of women treated with typical neuroleptics. J Clin Psychopharmacol 19:194–195, 1999

Corbacho AM, Martinez De La Escalera G, Clapp C: Roles of prolactin and related members of the prolactin/growth hormone/placental lactogen family in angiogenesis. J Endocrinol 173:219–238, 2002

Correa N, Opler LA, Kay SR: Amantadine in the treatment of neuroendocrine side effects of neuroleptics. J Clin Psychopharmacol 137:1117–1118, 1981

Costa D, Mestes E, Coban A: Breast and other cancer deaths in a mental hospital. Neoplasma 28:371–378, 1981

Crawford AMK, Beasley CM, Tollefson GD: The acute and long-term effect of olanzapine compared with placebo and haloperidol on serum prolactin concentrations. Schizophr Res 26:41–54, 1997

Curb JD, Hardy RJ, Labarthe DR, et al: Reserpine and breast cancer in the Hypertension Detection and Follow-up program. Hypertension 4:307–311, 1982

David SR, Taylor CC, Kinon BJ, et al: The effects of olanzapine, risperidone, and haloperidol on plasma prolactin levels in patients with schizophrenia. Clin Ther 22:1085–1096, 2000

Dickson RA, Dalby JT, Williams R, et al: Risperidone-induced prolactin elevations in premenopausal women with schizophrenia. Am J Psychiatry 12:1102–1103, 1995

Gazzola LR, Opler LA: Return of menstruation after switching from risperidone to olanzapine. J Clin Psychopharmacol 18:486–487, 1998

Ghadirian A, Chouinard G, Annabel L: Sexual dysfunction and plasma prolactin levels in neuroleptic treated schizophrenic outpatients. J Nerv Ment Dis 170:463–467, 1982

Gingell KH, Darley JS, Lengua CA, et al: Menstrual changes with antipsychotic drugs (letter). Br J Psychiatry 162:127, 1993

Gitlin MJ: Psychotropic medications and their effects on sexual function: diagnosis, biology, and treatment approaches. J Clin Psychiatry 55:406–413, 1994

Goff DC, Posever T, Herz L, et al: An exploratory haloperidol-controlled dose-finding study of ziprasidone in hospitalized patients with schizophrenia or schizoaffective disorder. J Clin Psychopharmacol 18:296–304, 1998

Goffin V, Touraine P, Pichard C, et al: Should prolactin be reconsidered as a therapeutic target in human breast cancer? Mol Cell Endocrinol 151:79–87, 1999

Goffin V, Binart N, Touraine P, et al: Prolactin: the new biology of an old hormone. Annu Rev Physiol 64:47–67, 2002

Goode DJ, Corbett WJ, Schey HM, et al: Breast cancer in hospitalized psychiatric patients. Am J Psychiatry 138:804–806, 1981

Grady D, Rueben SB, Pettiti DB, et al: Hormone therapy to prevent disease and prolong life in postmenopausal women. Ann Intern Med 117:1016–1037, 1992

Greenspan SL, Neer RM, Ridgeway EC, et al: Osteoporosis in men with hyperprolactinemic hypogonadism. Ann Intern Med 104:777–782, 1986

Halbreich U, Palter S: Accelerated osteoporosis in psychiatric patients: possible pathophysiological processes. Schizophr Bull 22:447–454, 1996

Halbreich U, Rojansky N, Palter S, et al: Decreased bone mineral density in medicated psychiatric patients. Psychosom Med 57:485–491, 1995

Halbreich U, Shen J, Panaro V: Are chronic psychiatric patients at increased risk for developing breast cancer? Am J Psychiatry 153:550–560, 1996

Hamner MB, Arvanitis LA, Miller BG, et al: Plasma prolactin in schizophrenia subjects treated with Seroquel (ICI 204,636). Psychopharmacol Bull 32:107–110, 1996

Hankinson SE, Willett WC, Michaud DS, et al: Plasma prolactin levels and subsequent risk of breast cancer in postmenopausal women. J Natl Cancer Inst 7:629–634, 1999

Harper ME, Peeling WB, Cowley T, et al: Plasma steroid and protein hormone concentration in patients with prostatic carcinoma, before and during estrogen therapy. Acta Endocrinol (Copenh) 81:409–426, 1976

Heinonen OP, Shapiro S, Tuominen L, et al: Reserpine use in relation to breast cancer. Lancet 2:675–677, 1974

Hellewell JSE: Antipsychotic tolerability: the attitudes and perceptions of medical professionals, patients and caregivers towards side effects of antipsychotic therapy. Eur Neuropsychopharmacol 8(suppl 1):24, 1998

Huber TJ, Rollnick J, Wilheims J, et al: Estradiol levels in psychotic disorders. Psychoneuroendocrinology 26:27–73, 2001

Hummer M, Kemmler G, Kurz M, et al: Sexual disturbances during clozapine and haloperidol treatment for schizophrenia. Am J Psychiatry 15:631–633, 1999

Ingram DM, Nottage EM, Roberts AN: Prolactin and breast cancer risk. Med J Aust 153:469–473, 1990

Inoue H, Hazama H, Ogura C: Neuroendocrinological study of amenorrhea induced by antipsychotics drugs (letter). Folia Psychiatr Neurol (Jpn) 34:191, 1980

Kane JM, Cooper TB, Sachar EJ et al: Clozapine: plasma levels and prolactin response. Psychopharmacology (Berl) 73:184–187, 1981

Kaneda Y, Fujii A: Effects of chronic neuroleptic administration on the hypothalamo-pituitary-gonadal axis of male schizophrenics. Prog Neuropsychopharmacol Biol Psychiatry 24:251–258, 2000

Kapur S, Seeman P: Does fast dissociation from the dopamine d(2) receptor explain the action of atypical antipsychotics? A new hypothesis. Am J Psychiatry 158:360–369, 2001

Kapur S, Langlois X, Vinken P, et al: The differential effects of atypical antipsychotics on prolactin elevation are explained by their differential blood-brain disposition: a pharmacological analysis in rats. J Pharmacol Exp Ther 302:1129–1134, 2002

Keeley EJ, Reiss JP, Drinkwater DT, et al: Bone mineral density, sex hormones, and long-term use of neuroleptic agent in men. Endocr Pract 3:209–213, 1997

Kim KS, Pae CU, Chae JH: Effects of olanzapine on prolactin levels of female patients with schizophrenia treated with risperidone. J Clin Psychiatry 63:408–413, 2002

Kim YK, Kim L, Lee MS: Risperidone and associated amenorrhea: a report of 5 cases. J Clin Psychiatry 60:315–317, 1999

Kleinberg DL, Davis JM, DeCoster R, et al: Prolactin levels and adverse events in patients treated with risperidone. J Clin Psychopharmacol 19:57–61, 1999

Klibanski A, Biller BM, Rosenthal DI, et al: Effects of prolactin and estrogen deficiency in amenorrheic bone loss. J Clin Endocrinol Metab 67:124–130, 1988

Kotin J, Wilbert DE, Verburg D, et al: Thioridazine and sexual dysfunction. Am J Psychiatry 133:82–85, 1976

Kuruvilla A, Peedicayil J, Srikrishna G, et al: A study of serum prolactin levels in schizophrenia: comparison of males and females. Clin Exp Pharmacol Physiol 19:603–606, 1992

Labarthe DR, O'Fallon LWM: Reserpine and breast cancer: a community-based longitudinal study of 2,000 hypertensive women. JAMA 243:2304–2310, 1980

Laska EM, Siegel C, Meisner M, et al: Matched pair study of reserpine use and breast cancer. Lancet 2:296–300, 1975

Llovera M, Touraine P, Kelly PA, et al: Involvement of prolactin in breast cancer: redefining the molecular targets. Exp Gerontol 35:41–51, 2000

Mack TM, Henderson BE, Gerkins VR, et al: Reserpine and breast cancer in a retirement community. N Engl J Med 292:1366–1371, 1975

Magharious W, Goff DC, Amico E: Relationship of gender and menstrual status to symptoms and medication side effects in patients with schizophrenia. Psychiatry Res 77:159–166, 1998

Markianos M, Hatzimanolis J, Lykouras L: Gonadal axis hormones in male schizophrenic patients during treatment with haloperidol and after switch to risperidone. Psychopharmacology (Berl) 143:270–272, 1999

Meltzer HY: Clinical studies on the mechanism of action of clozapine: the dopamine-serotonin hypothesis of schizophrenia. Psychopharmacology 99 (suppl): S18–S27, 1989

Meston CM, Frohlich PF: The neurobiology of sexual function. Arch Gen Psychiatry 57:1012–1030, 2000

Mortensen PB: Neuroleptic treatment and other factors modifying cancer risk in schizophrenic patients. Acta Psychiatr Scand 75:585–590, 1987

Mortensen PB: Neuroleptic medication and reduced risk of prostate cancer in schizophrenic patients. Acta Psychiatr Scand 85:390–393, 1992

Mortensen PB: The occurrence of cancer in first admitted schizophrenic patients. Schizophr Res 12:185–194, 1994

Neidhart M: Prolactin in autoimmune disease. Proc Soc Exp Biol Med 217:408–419, 1998

Perkins DO: Predictors of non-compliance in patients with schizophrenia. J Clin Psychiatry 63:1121–1128, 2002

Reiter E, Hennuy B, Bruyninx M, et al: Effects of pituitary hormones on the prostate. Prostate 38:159–165, 1999

Rinieris P, Hatzimanolis J, Markianos M, et al: Effects of treatment with various doses of haloperidol on the pituitary-gonadal axis in male schizophrenic patients. Neuropsychobiology 22:146–149, 1989

Rose DP, Pruitt BT: Plasma prolactin levels in patients with breast cancer. Cancer 48:2687–2691, 1981

Sandison RA, Whitelaw E, Currie JD: Clinical trials with Mellaril in the treatment of schizophrenia. Journal of Mental Sciences 106:732–741, 1960

Saroff J, Kirdani RY, Chu M, et al: Measurement of prolactin and androgens in patients with prostatic disease. Oncology 37:4–52, 1980

Schreiber S, Segman SH: Risperidone-induced galactorrhea. Psychopharmacologia 130:300–301, 1997

Seagraves RT: Effects of psychotropic drugs on human erection and ejaculation. Arch Gen Psychiatry 4:275–284, 1989

Secreto G, Recchione C, Cavalleri A, et al: Circulating levels of testosterone, 17ß-oestradiol, luteinising hormone and prolactin in postmenopausal breast cancer patients. Br J Cancer 47:269–275, 1983

Shader RI, Nahum JP, DiMascio A: Amenorrhea, in Psychotropic Drug Side Effects: Clinical and Theoretical Perspectives. Edited by Shader RI, DiMascio A. Baltimore, MD, Williams & Wilkins, 1970, pp 10–15

Shapiro S, Parsells JL, Rosenberg L, et al: Risk of breast cancer in relation to use of rauwolfia alkaloids. Eur J Clin Pharmacol 26:143–146, 1984

Shennan DB: Regulation of water and solute transport across mammalian plasma cell membranes by prolactin. J Dairy Res 61:155–166, 1994

Siever LJ: The effects of amantadine on prolactin levels and galactorrhea on neuroleptic-treated patients. J Clin Psychopharmacol 1:2–7, 1981

Siimes MA, Ropponen P, Aalberg V, et al: Prolactinemia in adolescent males surviving malignancies in childhood: impaired dating activity. J Adolesc Health 14:543–547, 1993

Siris SG, Siris ES, van Kammen DP, et al: Effects of dopamine blockade on gonadotropins and testosterone in men. Am J Psychiatry 137:211–214, 1980

Smith S, Wheeler MJ, Murray R, et al: The effect of antipsychotic induced hyperprolactinemia on the hypothalamic-pituitary-gonadal axis. J Clin Psychopharmacol 22:109–114, 2002

Stanford JL, Martin EJ, Brinton LA, et al: Rauwolfia use and breast cancer: a case-control study. J Natl Cancer Inst 76:817–822, 1986

Turrone P, Kapur S, Seeman MV, et al: Elevation of prolactin by atypical antipsychotics. Am J Psychiatry 159:133–135, 2002

Valevski A, Modai I, Zbarski E, et al: Effect of amantadine on sexual dysfunction in neuroleptic-treated male schizophrenic patients. Clin Neuropharmacol 21:355–357, 1998

Wang DY, De Stavola BL, Bulbrook RD, et al: Relationship of blood prolactin levels and the risk of subsequent breast cancer. Int J Epidemiol 21: 214–221, 1992

Wennbo H, Tornell J: The role of prolactin and growth hormone in breast cancer. Oncogene 19:1072–1076, 2000

Wesselmann U, Windgassen K: Galactorrhea: subjective response by schizophrenic patients. Acta Psychiatr Scand 91:152–155, 1995

Windgassen K, Wellelmann U, Schulze M, et al: Galactorrhea and hyperprolactinemia in schizophrenic patients on neuroleptics: frequency and etiology. Neuropsychobiology 33:142–146, 1996

Winters SJ, Troen P: Altered pulsatile secretion of lueteinizing hormone in hypogonadal men with hyperprolactinaemia. Clin Endocrinol 21:257–263, 1984

Writing Group for the Women's Health Initiative Investigators: Risks and benefits of estrogen plus progestin in healthy postmenopausal women: principal results from the Women's Health Initiative randomized controlled trial. JAMA 17:321–333, 2002

Wudarsky M, Nicolson R, Hamburger SD, et al: Elevated prolactin in pediatric patients on typical and atypical antipsychotics. J Child Adolesc Psychopharmacol 9:239–245, 1999

Yu-Lee LY: Prolactin modulation of immune and inflammatory responses. Recent Prog Horm Res 57:435–455, 2002

Index

Italic page numbers indicate text within tables or figures.

616
Med

Medical illness and
schizophrenia.

DATE			
7/13/06		7/29/14	
2/28/12	11/25/14	4/2/15	
7/14/12		2/21/17	
7/20/12			
7/30/13			
10/29/13			